SKIPPER'S MEDICAL EMERGENCY HANDBOOK

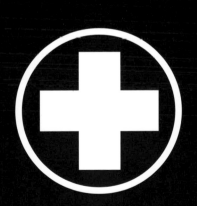

SECOND EDITION

ADLARD COLES
Bloomsbury Publishing Plc
50 Bedford Square, London, WC1B 3DP, UK

BLOOMSBURY, ADLARD COLES and the Adlard Coles logo are trademarks of
Bloomsbury Publishing Plc

First published in Great Britain 2008
This edition published 2018

Authors: Dr Spike Briggs and Dr Campbell Mackenzie

Conceived, edited and designed by Quarto Publishing plc,
an imprint of The Quarto Group
The Old Brewery, 6 Blundell Street, London N7 9BH, UK
www.quartoknows.com

A catalogue record for this book is available from the British Library

Library of Congress Cataloguing-in-Publication data has been applied for

ISBN: PB: 978-1-4729-6020-7; ePub: 978-1-4729-6019-1;
ePDF: 978-1-4729-6021-4

2 4 6 8 10 9 7 5 3 1

Typeset in ITC Franklin Gothic
Printed in China

Bloomsbury Publishing Plc makes every effort to ensure that the papers used in
the manufacture of our books are natural, recyclable products made from wood
grown in well-managed forests. Our manufacturing processes conform to the
environmental regulations of the country of origin.

To find out more about our authors and books visit www.bloomsbury.com and sign
up for our newsletters

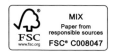

SKIPPER'S MEDICAL EMERGENCY HANDBOOK

FIRST AID AT SEA

SECOND EDITION

CONTENTS

CONTENTS CONTINUED

INTRODUCTION

Remote, isolated oceans provide the ultimate wilderness in which to practice medicine. More and more yachts – single-handed, double-handed, or fully crewed and perhaps carrying children – are venturing into these watery wildernesses. Whether you are racing, cruising, or working at sea, a good degree of self-sufficiency is essential, and never more so than when faced with medical crises. Therefore, a vessel venturing beyond the immediate range of helicopter rescue must be prepared to cope with all its own medical problems.

This emergency handbook provides a *vade-mecum*, literally a "take with you" reference book that will answer the burning question when faced with a sick or traumatized sailor, "What do I do?" For the yacht or ship with an on-board medic of some experience, it will act as an aide-memoire for recalling medical knowledge, while reassuring and confirming that the correct action is being taken.

The phrase "Common things happen most commonly" applies equally to injuries and illnesses, both on land and at sea. Therefore, this handbook concentrates on the sort of simple, minor problems you are most likely to encounter at sea and supplies the basic information on what to do, with simple, easy-to-follow illustrations on how to do it. The handbook will supplement what expertise is available on board, helping you to make the correct diagnosis and administer the most appropriate treatment. It also gives guidance on assessing the severity of medical problems, outlining whether the casualty should be managed on board, landed, or evacuated at sea.

Importantly, the handbook also reinforces the message that anticipation of medical emergencies will avert trouble later. In medicine there is a well-known saying that "An ounce of prevention is worth a pound of treatment." Parts of this book, particularly the section on preparation and planning, should be read prior to leaving port, as they contain essential information that should be absorbed before you get on board.

If the crew can avoid going overboard, being struck on the head by the boom, or falling below deck, serious problems are, fortunately, remarkably uncommon. However, boats can injure people. Bad weather may hasten the onset of medical problems and will invariably make injuries and illnesses appear more serious than they really are. It is undoubtedly more difficult to treat casualties on a wildly pitching boat, surrounded by seasick crew, than it is on land.

The crew will have faith in the capabilities of their skipper or on-board medic. They will expect that the medic can get them out of immediate trouble and safeguard them for as long as it takes to either recover or reach professional help, should it be necessary. However, confidence does not always reflect competence. Therefore, it is essential that the captain and the crew member deputed as on-board medic both obtain suitable medical training and certification; this is equally as important as their equivalent seagoing qualification.

When spray peppers the cockpit like buckshot, solid water sweeps the deck, and the boat's motion is erratic and nauseating, breakages occur, equipment fails, and great demands are made on the crew. It is at this highly inconvenient time that injuries are most likely to occur. These are the situations when your emergency handbook will be immensely useful, making it an essential part of the on-board library. It will be invaluable when faced with a casualty, whatever the position of the yacht, especially when it is difficult to establish communications with shore.

Remember that seeking medical advice is one of the most important actions to take when faced with a difficult medical problem. A healthy ship is a happy ship, and above all, the ultimate goal of on-board medics is to save and preserve lives.

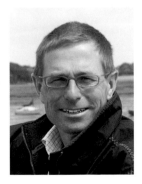

Spike Briggs

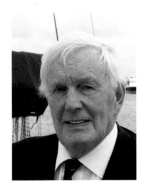

Campbell Mackenzie

HOW TO USE THIS BOOK

This book is divided into five chapters and within those into indivdual entries. Before you depart, read the Preparation chapter, where you will learn how to equip the boat and make ready the medic and crew. At sea, the chapter you choose will depend on the circumstances: Emergency Care: How to Save and Preserve Life; Trauma and Accidents; or Medical Disorders. All three of these chapters will refer you to the final chapter, Emergency Medical Procedures, where you will find step-by-step instructions on making vital assessments, performing minor wound repair, stabilizing injuries, and carrying out emergency procedures.

The Emergencies, Trauma, and Disorders chapters all use a similar format. Within the appropriate entry, consult the flow chart for a condensed summary of evaluation and treatment. The remainder of the entry will expand on this outline, further explaining what to look for in your examination, giving hints on prevention, and describing the features of specific injuries and treatments.

Red boxes emphasize emergency actions

Red arrows indicate severe risks and emergency responses

Follow cross-references to further detail or to systematic instructions

Emergency procedures are explained using step-by-step ilustrations

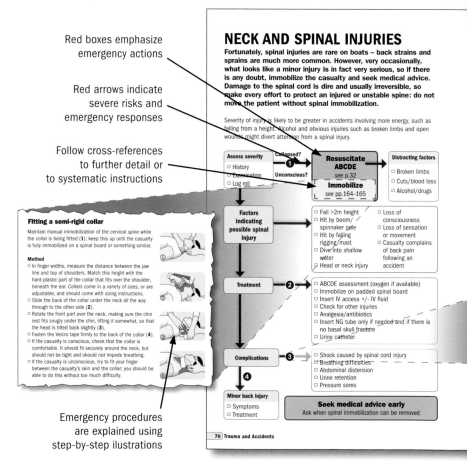

NECK AND SPINAL INJURIES

Fortunately, spinal injuries are rare on boats – back strains and sprains are much more common. However, very occasionally, what looks like a minor injury is in fact very serious, so if there is any doubt, immobilize the casualty and seek medical advice. Damage to the spinal cord is dire and usually irreversible, so make every effort to protect an injured or unstable spine: do not move the patient without spinal immobilization.

Severity of injury is likely to be greater in accidents involving more energy, such as falling from a height. Alcohol and obvious injuries such as broken limbs and open wounds might divert attention from a spinal injury.

Assess severity
- History
- Examination
- Log roll

Collapsed? ➊
Unconscious?

Resuscitate ABCDE
see p.32
Immobilize
see pp.164–165

Distracting factors
- Broken limbs
- Cuts/blood loss
- Alcohol/drugs

Factors indicating possible spinal injury
- Fall >2m height
- Hit by boom/ spinnaker pole
- Hit by falling rigging/mast
- Dive into shallow water
- Head or neck injury
- Loss of consciousness
- Loss of sensation or movement
- Casualty complains of back pain following an accident

Treatment ➋
- ABCDE assessment (oxygen if available)
- Immobilize on padded spinal board
- Insert IV access +/- IV fluid
- Check for other injuries
- Analgesia/antibiotics
- Insert NG tube only if needed and if there is no basal skull fracture
- Urine catheter

Complications ➌
- Shock caused by spinal cord injury
- Breathing difficulties
- Abdominal distension
- Urine retention
- Pressure sores

➍

Minor back injury
- Symptoms
- Treatment

Seek medical advice early
Ask when spinal immobilization can be removed

Fitting a semi-rigid collar

Maintain manual immobilization of the cervical spine while the collar is being fitted (**1**); keep this up until the casualty is fully immobilized on a spinal board or something similar.

Method
- In finger widths, measure the distance between the jaw line and top of shoulders. Match this height with the hard-plastic part of the collar that fits over the shoulder, beneath the ear. Collars come in a variety of sizes, or are adjustable, and should come with sizing instructions.
- Slide the back of the collar under the neck all the way through to the other side (**2**).
- Rotate the front part over the neck, making sure the chin rest fits snugly under the chin, lifting it somewhat, so that the head is tilted back slightly (**3**).
- Fasten the Velcro tape firmly to the back of the collar (**4**).
- If the casualty is conscious, check that the collar is comfortable. It should fit securely around the neck, but should not be too tight and should not impede breathing.
- If the casualty is unconscious, try to fit your finger between the casualty's skin and the collar; you should be able to do this without too much difficulty.

ACRONYMS AND SYMBOLS USED IN THIS BOOK

ABC	Airway, Breathing, Circulation	see p.30
ABCDE	Approach, Assess, Airway; Breathing; Circulation; Disability; Environment	see p.32
AED	Automated External Defibrillator	see p.161
AVPU	Alert; Vocal stimuli provoke response; Painful stimuli provoke response; Unresponsive	see p.168
BLS	Basic Life Support	see p.30
bpm	beats per minute	
EPIRB	Emergency Position-Indicating Radio Beacon	
GCS	Glasgow Coma Score	see p.169
IM (injections)	Intramuscular	
IV (fluids)	Intravenous	
NG (tube)	Nasogastric	
NSAIDs	Nonsteroidal Anti-inflammatory Drugs	
<	Less than	
>	Greater than	

---

❶ History and examination

- ABCDE assessment (see p.32) takes priority over everything else.
- Anyone with a head injury may well have a spinal injury as well.
- A proper examination for possible neck and spinal injuries will require a log roll (see p.163), which requires four people to turn the casualty and one to examine the back.

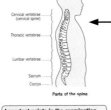

Cervical vertebrae
(cervical spine)

Thoracic vertebrae

Lumbar vertebrae

Sacrum

Coccyx

Parts of the spine

Anatomical illustrations provide a guide to major parts of the body, to help you when reporting to on-shore medical support

Important points in the history	**Important points in the examination**

□ How did the accident happen?
 □ Where is the pain?
 □ Are there any symptoms of nerve damage?
     – pins and needles
     – loss of movement
 – numbness
 □ Any previous history of back pain or injuries?
	Look Obvious injuries to head, neck, spine; swelling, bruising
	 Feel Tenderness, steps in spine, can the casualty feel touch and pain?
	 Move Can patient move body and limbs? If neck injured, do not move it
	 Document Tone, power, sensation for all limbs and the main body

Quick-reference lists explain what you need to find out from the casualty and what to look for during an examination

❷ Treatment

A casualty with a suspected spinal injury must be evacuated as soon as possible.
Immobilization (see pp.164–165) The whole body must be immobilized as effectively as possible using a neck collar and a padded board.
IV access and fluid Casualty may have low blood pressure and need IV fluid.
Nasogastric (NG) tube, urinary catheter (see pp.186–88) An immobilized patient may be kept hydrated by an NG tube and will need a urinary catheter.
Analgesia, antibiotics Pain relief to settle the casualty; antibiotics for an open wound.

❸ Complications

- Low blood pressure (shock) may be caused by relaxation of blood vessels due to spinal cord damage. Seek medical advice about how much fluid to give.
- If the spinal cord injury is high in the chest or in the neck, the casualty may not be able to breathe properly. This is an ominous problem on a boat. Give oxygen if available and follow ABC assessment if the patient stops breathing (see p.30).
- The gut may stop working, and the casualty may vomit. Once an NG tube is in place, aspirate all the stomach contents out initially to reduce the risk.

❹ Minor back injuries

Symptoms A minor back injury will cause localized pain that is worse on straining or coughing. Pain may extend down the leg (sciatica) and posture may be abnormal.
Treatments Administer pain relief to allow mobilization and prevent stiffness. If the casualty has sciatica, advise rest and seek medical advice. Care should be taken with the posture during vigorous activities such as winching and helming.

A numbering system helps you quickly locate more detail on such subjects as complications, specific injuries or disorders, and signs of severe conditions

Neck and Spinal Injuries **76**

Preparation

INITIAL CONSIDERATIONS IN PLANNING THE VOYAGE

Planning a voyage requires time, knowledge, experience, and careful attention to detail. If you are lacking in any of these areas, get help and advice from someone who has the necessary expertise. Planning medical resources and shore support is a specialized and essential part of this process. If the worst event happens, planning is irrevocably over, and action must begin. Unless proper planning has been undertaken, the action you take may be inappropriate and could endanger life and limb.

There are a number of main areas, considered below, that affect the medical planning for any voyage, whether it is a sprint around the cans on a cold winter's day, cruising the Caribbean, or an exploratory voyage to the polar regions.

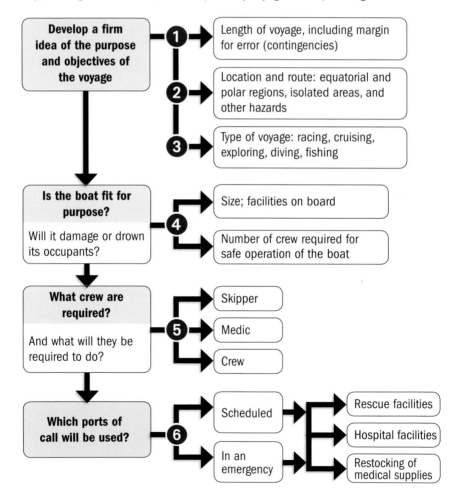

Develop a firm idea of the purpose and objectives of the voyage

1. Length of voyage, including margin for error (contingencies)
2. Location and route: equatorial and polar regions, isolated areas, and other hazards
3. Type of voyage: racing, cruising, exploring, diving, fishing

Is the boat fit for purpose?
Will it damage or drown its occupants?

4. Size; facilities on board
   Number of crew required for safe operation of the boat

What crew are required?
And what will they be required to do?

5. Skipper
   Medic
   Crew

Which ports of call will be used?

6. Scheduled
   In an emergency

   Rescue facilities
   Hospital facilities
   Restocking of medical supplies

❶ Length of voyage

The length of time you will spend at sea will determine the amount and type of medical supplies you will require. The longer the voyage, the greater the complexity of medical conditions that may require treatment. Longer voyages therefore generally require fitter crew with fewer pre-existing medical conditions and more comprehensive medical support, both on board and on shore. Contingencies must be built in for unforeseen events and accidents that might significantly prolong the voyage.

❷ Location and route

The availability of medical support and rescue facilities reduces rapidly as a route moves away from inhabited land and the working range of coastguard helicopters. Some oceanic areas, such as the North Atlantic, are busy with commercial traffic, which may be a source of medical aid. Others, such as the Southern Ocean, are some of the last true wildernesses of the world, where rescue may be weeks away. Routes that venture into the polar and equatorial regions bring special climatic medical risks. Certain ports of call, such as those in malarial regions, may pose particular risks.

❸ Type of voyage

Racing involves increased risk of trauma as the boat is driven forwards to the boundary of control and sometimes beyond it. Cruising may be less directly injurious, but the crew may be older and have more pre-existing medical conditions. Diving offers special risks of barotrauma, decompression sickness, and gas problems.

❹ The boat

It should be common sense that the boat is fit for its purpose, but there are many records of boats first injuring and then drowning their occupants. From the medical point of view, it is worth considering: how an injured crew member would be evacuated below deck or to a helicopter; where simple "medical procedures" may be performed safely; and where the medical kit and grab bag should be stored for rapid access in an emergency. Larger boats have the advantage of having dedicated space and weight-carrying capacity for medical activities and stores.

❺ The crew

Routes that are particularly rigorous or remote, as well as long distances and extreme climates, require fit crew and comprehensive medical training for the skipper and medic. Short-handed crew work harder and become more exhausted, and consequently incur more injuries and illnesses. Medical screening of crew may be necessary. It is crucial to appoint a suitable medic, who will support the captain in dealing with medical problems on board. Both captain and medic must be thoroughly up-to-date on any medical issues in case the other becomes injured.

❻ Ports of call

All possible ports of call should be identified, either as scheduled stopovers or for use in an emergency. Their facilities for rescue, definitive care, and medical resupply require consideration.

TASKS BEFORE DEPARTURE

Many tasks require your attention prior to departure, including fitting out, taking safety measures, victualing, and checking charts and weather faxes. However, thought must also be given to the crew's health and welfare, an area that is often given low priority in the work schedule. Such planning may well dictate the success or failure of the trip. Crew should be able to feel confident that, should they be struck down, treatment on board will be the best available under the circumstances.

Careful attention to the previous section (Initial Considerations in Planning the Voyage) will highlight the tasks that must be completed prior to departure. This is the time to find answers to your questions, when you can consult the experts while you are warm and dry and not in fear for your own or fellow crew's safety.

Crew selection

Sailing in remote areas is no longer the preserve of the young and fit. A crew should, however, be generally physically fit prior to the voyage, with particular attention paid to cardiopulmonary fitness and lower-limb strength, both of which will decline when crew are confined on board a yacht. It is worth advising the crew on matters of well-being, hygiene, healthy nutrition, and physical fitness in good time before departure.

There is a relatively high risk involved in taking crew who are dependent on oral medication for life-threatening conditions, such as organ transplant, epilepsy, and heart disease. Insulin-dependent diabetes mellitus and severe asthma also involve greater risk offshore. Stringent exclusion criteria should be applied to voyages beyond helicopter range and might exclude crew with any of these conditions.

Medical screening may take the form of a self-declaration questionnaire (*see* pp.198–99), with or without confirmation by the family doctor, or it may involve a formal physical examination and testing. Such screening will appear onerous but will avoid potentially serious complications, which may endanger the whole boat.

Selection of the medic

Who makes the best medic? Ideally, the person should be well motivated to undertake the task, and it helps if he or she has some sort of medical, dental, or veterinary background or some experience of first aid. Doctors, ambulance workers, nurses, firefighters, and police officers are highly suitable candidates. People working in these environments appreciate the importance of compassion, confidentiality, communication, and documentation. Once a suitable person has been identified, he or she should be given responsibility regarding the past medical history of the crew and should be involved in ordering the medical kit.

Training should be undertaken by both the medic and skipper. Special training in the particular conditions that may be encountered at sea, such as prolonged immersion, drowning, and hypothermia, is essential.

Immunization

All crew must undergo an immunization update program for all those areas that may be visited during the course of the voyage. Information on these requirements is easily available from either a family doctor or from a range of online sources (*see* p.204 for a list of immunization requirements in various parts of the world).

Medical kit

The medical kit could be vital to keeping an injured or sick crew member alive. For an explanation of the different types of kits available and the principles underlying the design, content, location, and maintenance of an effective kit, *see* pp.20–23; for sample kit lists, *see* pp.205–207.

Communication and medical support

The universal advice in all medical emergencies is to **seek medical advice early** (telemedical support). This is only possible if working communication equipment is available and the sources of advice are known in advance. Means of communication must be reliable. For short-range communications, VHF radio may be the best option, or even mobile telephone! More distant communications may require a satellite system, using email or voice communication, or the Inmarsat-C™ messaging system. Telemedicine is increasingly common but may require video transmission and reception as well as medical expertise to interpret the images.

Shore support for medical emergencies is made possible via international maritime rescue coordination centres (MRCC) and other such organizations that provide support for expeditions to remote places. Those involved in larger expeditions may wish to organize their own shore medical support team, which can then be tailored to the crew's specific requirements.

Ports of call

The facilities at all possible ports of call, either scheduled or identified for use in emergency, should be investigated. Rescue facilities may or may not be available, and local hospital care may offer variable services. Crew should be made aware of the particular risks a port of call may pose. An up-to-date pilot book is essential. The Internet is, of course, also an excellent source of information.

Restocking of medical supplies may be problematic, especially if the local language is not English. However, most drugs are available in most places, albeit in different packaging and using different trade names. The generic names, however, should remain consistent around the world. Arrangements may be made to ship resupply items from home, but this may require customs clearance.

Insurance

Insurance must cover not only medical treatment but also the possible cost of rescue, which may be considerable. The medic on the boat may not be covered to treat crew in the territorial waters or ports of call of certain countries. He or she may be open to legal action if some treatment inadvertently causes harm. Insurance companies may require the medical details of all crew.

ON-BOARD EMERGENCY PROCEDURES AND CREW ROLES

At sea, as in other areas of life, prevention is always better and easier than a cure. Good planning of ocean voyages, based on risk assessment, will allow effective treatment of on-board emergencies, by ensuring anticipation of the expected and an ability to cope with the unexpected. A proactive crew will always out-perform a reactive one.

It is said that "No plan survives first contact with the enemy." If the captain and vessel medic are disabled by an accident, their roles will have to be taken over by other first-aid trained crew. Rigid procedural planning is therefore best replaced by a simple, generic format that addresses the most common medical emergencies and can be easily followed.

Dealing with medical emergencies is a continual learning process, and, as with man overboard drills, practice in the management of simulated on-board casualties should be part of all work–up training sails. Medical planning will depend on the medical capabilities of the crew (you may be lucky enough to have a doctor or other medical professionals in the team) and the underlying medical problems presented by the crew. Every new crew member should be briefed on emergency medical procedures; this is absolutely essential to ensure the best outcome when and if disaster strikes.

The aims of dealing with medical emergencies at sea are to:

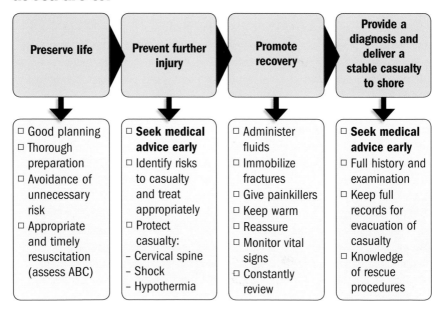

Preserve life	Prevent further injury	Promote recovery	Provide a diagnosis and deliver a stable casualty to shore
☐ Good planning ☐ Thorough preparation ☐ Avoidance of unnecessary risk ☐ Appropriate and timely resuscitation (assess ABC)	☐ **Seek medical advice early** ☐ Identify risks to casualty and treat appropriately ☐ Protect casualty: – Cervical spine – Shock – Hypothermia	☐ Administer fluids ☐ Immobilize fractures ☐ Give painkillers ☐ Keep warm ☐ Reassure ☐ Monitor vital signs ☐ Constantly review	☐ **Seek medical advice early** ☐ Full history and examination ☐ Keep full records for evacuation of casualty ☐ Knowledge of rescue procedures

General procedure for on-board medical emergencies

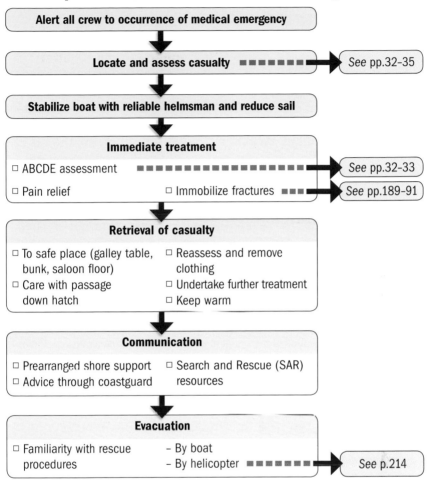

Alert all crew to occurrence of medical emergency

↓

Locate and assess casualty ━━━━━━━━▶ *See pp.32–35*

↓

Stabilize boat with reliable helmsman and reduce sail

↓

Immediate treatment

☐ ABCDE assessment ━━━━━━━━━━━━━━▶ *See pp.32–33*

☐ Pain relief ☐ Immobilize fractures ━━━▶ *See pp.189–91*

↓

Retrieval of casualty

☐ To safe place (galley table, bunk, saloon floor)
☐ Care with passage down hatch
☐ Reassess and remove clothing
☐ Undertake further treatment
☐ Keep warm

↓

Communication

☐ Prearranged shore support
☐ Advice through coastguard
☐ Search and Rescue (SAR) resources

↓

Evacuation

☐ Familiarity with rescue procedures
– By boat
– By helicopter ━━━━━━━━▶ *See p.214*

Crew roles

Captain Overall management and preplanning. In an emergency, try to avoid getting involved, but remain briefed on progress. Plan ahead, in case evacuation or landing become necessary.

Helm Control the boat, ensuring a stable and safe working platform: there should be no waves on deck and no accidental gybes, or sudden manoeuvres.

Medic Assess and safely retrieve the casualty. Avoid becoming injured yourself. Always seek medical advice early and liaise with the captain to ensure a coordinated response.

Navigator Know where you are and where you are going, and be prepared to transmit this information to the local rescue authorities.

Watch leader Call all hands on deck if necessary and let members of the watch handle the casualty if appropriate.

Other crew Stand by to help with treating the casualty, sailing the boat, and preparing the casualty for evacuation.

MEDICAL KIT DESIGN – WHAT IS NEEDED

Medical kit design depends on several factors, but the most important are the guidelines issued by the local regulatory authorities, which must be adhered to by all boats that come under their jurisdiction. Usually, the contents of the kit may be varied, under medical guidance, taking into account the size and purpose of the boat. For instance, small yachts may not be required to carry body bags and stretchers. The guidelines are generally more comprehensive the further the voyage ventures from land and are at their most extensive for those voyages that take the vessel beyond helicopter range (categories include coastal, offshore, and ocean). For sample kit lists, see pp.206–207.

Whoever is going to be the medic on board must be involved in ordering the medical kit, so they know what is in there and how to use it. There is no point in taking something like a defibrillator if no one on board knows what to do with it. The contents and quantities of the medical kit must take into account:

□ Duration of the expedition

□ Number of crew

□ Type of voyage
  – Racing is obviously more inherently dangerous than cruising

□ Proposed route
  – The more remote, the greater the need for self-sufficiency

□ Medical expertise on board
  – If you have a doctor on board, a more sophisticated kit may be justifiable

□ Medical history of the crew members
  – Older crew may have more medical problems
  – Special consideration for: heart disease, asthma, epilepsy, diabetes, allergies

□ Opportunities for resupply in ports of call
  – Generally, English-speaking countries are easier for resupply. Trade names vary in other countries, but generic names should remain recognizable.

Medicines and medical hardware are expensive and various items in a kit become out-of-date regularly, so thorough checks before departure should be made to ensure the kit is fit-for-purpose. All medical manuals, charts, and documentation must accompany the kit. Storage of the kit is also crucial: It must be in a safe place, but on the other hand must be instantly accessible if it is needed in an emergency. Keep kits dry and store them off the boat when not in use. Standard medical kits can be obtained from suppliers, who may also supply custom kits, under medical guidance.

The principles behind a successful medical kit

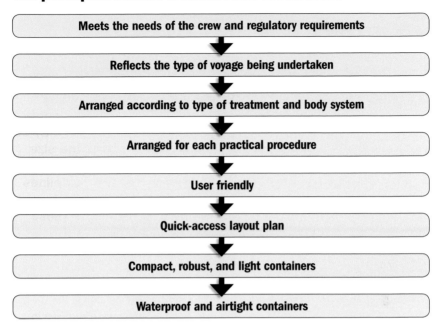

Meets the needs of the crew and regulatory requirements

↓

Reflects the type of voyage being undertaken

↓

Arranged according to type of treatment and body system

↓

Arranged for each practical procedure

↓

User friendly

↓

Quick-access layout plan

↓

Compact, robust, and light containers

↓

Waterproof and airtight containers

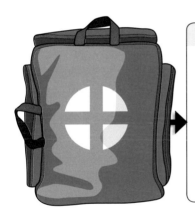

Separate stores bag

A separate stores bag can carry items that do not fit into the "body system" scheme (see p.23).

Contents might include:
- ☐ IV fluid (if carried)
- ☐ Emergency/resuscitation drugs
- ☐ Defibrillator/airway equipment
- ☐ Hardware

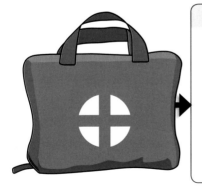

Basic first aid kit

A basic first aid kit will include items that can be used by any member of the crew.

Contents might include:
- ☐ Painkillers
- ☐ Cold, flu, and seasickness medications
- ☐ Adhesive bandages, simple dressings
- ☐ Sunscreen

HOW TO PUT A MEDICAL KIT TOGETHER

A medical kit could well contain several hundred items, and finding the right piece of equipment shouldn't become like the proverbial needle and haystack. Organization of the kit into sections is the key.

A good, systematic way of designing a comprehensive kit is to go though each body system (such as heart, gut, and skin), thinking about the common problems that happen on board and making sure that appropriate drugs, dressings, and hardware are included in the kit. All the medicines, hardware, needles, and so on for each body system should then be arranged into transparent, sealable bags or boxes, each with a laminated contents list. There should be separate bags, which do not fit into the "body system" scheme, containing: emergency drugs, including drugs for resuscitation; any hardware; IV and intramuscular drugs, with needles and syringes; IV fluid, if you have decided to carry it; and a defibrillator and airway equipment (again, this may not be considered necessary for all voyages).

This arrangement is illustrated opposite, with content suggestions for each section. All this equipment generally can't fit into one bag or box, especially for more comprehensive medical kits. A convenient way to arrange the overall kit is to use the following arrangement, loosely based on how often the parts of kit may be required:

First aid kit (to be kept in the saloon and to be used by any of the crew)

- Simple painkillers (such as paracetamol and ibuprofen)
- Adhesive bandages
- Sore throat lozenges
- Sunscreen
- Seasickness medications

Grab bag (for the life raft if abandoning ship; may also double as emergency treatment bag – see pp.206–207 for a sample list)

- Emergency analgesics (oral, intramuscular, suppositories)
- Seasickness medications (a large stock)
- Antibiotics
- Rehydration salts
- Suturing kit
- Splints, strapping, bandages

Medium-sized bag (frequently used items)

- Body system bags or boxes
- Emergency resuscitation kit
- First aid books, medical reference manuals

Large store bag (containing large, heavy equipment, not used often)

- Large splints
- IV fluid
- Stiff neck collars
- Stores of medicines for replenishment
- Oxygen cylinder/concentrator
- Defibrillator

Systematic arrangement for medical kit

First aid/seasickness
- Two types of anti-seasickness tablets
- Adhesive bandages
- Simple painkillers
- Sunscreen

Skin repair
- Sutures
- Skin stapler
- Antiseptic fluid
- Adhesive skin tape
- Skin glue

Painkillers
- Painkillers for mild, moderate, and severe pain
- Tablets, suppositories
- Injectable painkillers
- Local anaesthetics

Gut
- Laxatives
- Antidiarrhoeals
- Anti-indigestion
- Antispasmodics
- Rehydration salts

Emergency/allergies
- Adrenaline
- Steroids
- Antihistamines
- Sedatives
- Antiburn treatments

Trauma
- Splints
- Cast kits
- Strapping
- Dressings
- Bandages

Ear, nose, mouth, eyes
- Eye drops for pain
- Eye bath and shades
- Antibiotic eye and ear drops
- Dental kit

Infections
Antibiotics:
- Three types, in order to avoid allergies
- Oral and injectable antibiotics

TAKING A HISTORY FROM A CREW MEMBER

The first step in finding out what is wrong with the injured or sick crew member is to understand what has happened, both the immediate events and those further back in the past. This is no easy task, even on land in a hospital, and is particularly difficult at sea.

It is vital to remember that resuscitation and treatment of life-threatening injuries or illnesses takes precedence over a detailed history. However, a history of sorts is still absolutely necessary in emergency circumstances. The way to go about this is detailed in Assessment of a Sick or Injured Crew Member (*see* pp.32–35).

It is useful to have a structure for taking a history, both for medics and nonmedics; this will minimize the chances of essential information being missed. It also helps when transmitting medical information to shore, ensuring it is logical and comprehensive. Avoid medical jargon, which may be misleading if not used correctly. It is usually impossible to get the whole history in one go; it may come together over a few hours or even days, with information coming from any possible source, not just the casualty themselves.

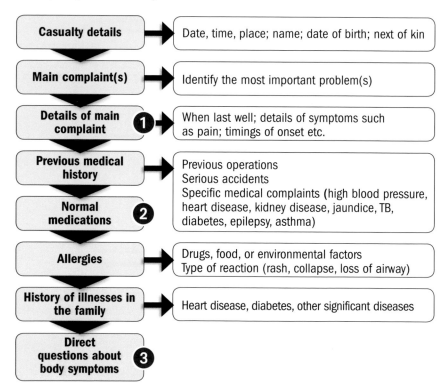

Casualty details	Date, time, place; name; date of birth; next of kin
Main complaint(s)	Identify the most important problem(s)
Details of main complaint ❶	When last well; details of symptoms such as pain; timings of onset etc.
Previous medical history	Previous operations Serious accidents Specific medical complaints (high blood pressure, heart disease, kidney disease, jaundice, TB, diabetes, epilepsy, asthma)
Normal medications ❷	
Allergies	Drugs, food, or environmental factors Type of reaction (rash, collapse, loss of airway)
History of illnesses in the family	Heart disease, diabetes, other significant diseases
Direct questions about body symptoms ❸	

❶ Details of main complaint

Complaint

What happened?	When were you last well?
What is wrong now?	Have you had this before?
When did you have it?	How long did it last?
Do you know what it is?	What treatment worked last time?

Pain

Where is the pain worst?	How severe is the pain (out of 10)?
Do you feel it anywhere else?	What makes it worse?
Is a sharp, dull, or constant?	What makes it better?

❷ Normal medications

- ☐ Specifically ask about heart medications, inhalers, epileptic and diabetic medications, antimalarials, oral contraceptives.
- ☐ Get details of immunizations, prophylactic medications, foreign travel.
- ☐ Also, ask about alternative medicines, homeopathic remedies, recreational drugs, alcohol, and smoking.

❸ Direct questions about body symptoms

Heart and circulation
Chest pain
Palpitations
Shortness of breath
Swelling of the ankles
Pain in the legs when walking

Lungs
Shortness of breath
Pain related to breathing
Cough
Wheeze
Sputum – amount and colour

Mouth, throat, and intestines
Nausea and vomiting
Indigestion
Abdominal pain
Distension
Last bowel movement – consistency?
Nature of stool – colour, blood?
Appetite, weight loss

Kidneys, bladder, and genitals
Pain on passing urine
Passing large volumes of urine frequently
Colour of urine
Loin pain
Discharge from genitals
Date of last menstrual period?
Any miscarriages?

Nervous system
Headache/stiff neck
Pain at looking at light
Visual acuity
Hearing
Fitting and fainting
Weakness or numbness in limbs

Musculoskeletal system/Skin
Pain or stiffness on moving limbs
Muscle pains or swelling
Joint pain or swelling
Stability while walking
Skin diseases/problems
Skin allergic reactions

EXAMINING A CREW MEMBER

A thorough examination is the second diagnostic stage. Examination may be difficult on-board, especially when the crew member is badly injured and fully clothed in foul-weather gear. It is worthwhile working out how to transfer an injured casualty from deck to below before having to do it.

Examination is a sensitive activity but is essential if the casualty is seriously injured or sick. The examination can be confined to the leg, if that is the only injured part, but it should be comprehensive, covering the whole body (including the back) if the casualty has fallen from a height and is unconscious. It may be necessary to expose part or all of the body, depending on the extent of injury. This may not only be inconvenient and difficult to achieve with a sick or injured casualty, it may also be detrimental, because the casualty could become very cold while uncovered. Minimizing the exposure time, and making best use of it, is imperative. The basis for examination is **look**, **feel**, **listen**, **move**, and compare left with right.

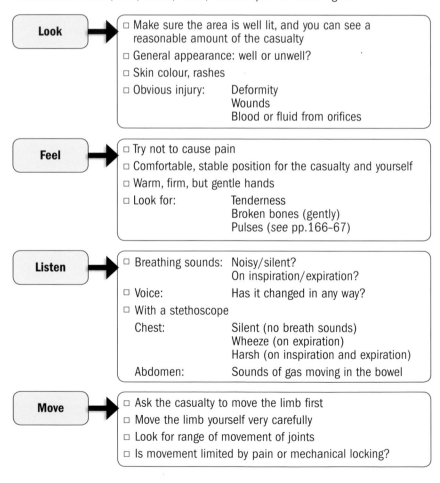

Look
- □ Make sure the area is well lit, and you can see a reasonable amount of the casualty
- □ General appearance: well or unwell?
- □ Skin colour, rashes
- □ Obvious injury: Deformity
                        Wounds
                        Blood or fluid from orifices

Feel
- □ Try not to cause pain
- □ Comfortable, stable position for the casualty and yourself
- □ Warm, firm, but gentle hands
- □ Look for: Tenderness
                  Broken bones (gently)
                  Pulses (see pp.166–67)

Listen
- □ Breathing sounds: Noisy/silent?
                       On inspiration/expiration?
- □ Voice: Has it changed in any way?
- □ With a stethoscope
       Chest: Silent (no breath sounds)
                       Wheeze (on expiration)
                       Harsh (on inspiration and expiration)
       Abdomen: Sounds of gas moving in the bowel

Move
- □ Ask the casualty to move the limb first
- □ Move the limb yourself very carefully
- □ Look for range of movement of joints
- □ Is movement limited by pain or mechanical locking?

Values for the adult body's vital signs

Vital sign	Normal range	Seriously unwell
Pulse (beats/minute)	50-100	<45 or >130
Systolic blood pressure (mmHg)	100-140	<80
Skin blanch test (capillary refill test, see p. 167)	<2 secs	>4 secs
Breathing rate (breaths per minute)	10-20	<8 or >25
Temperature (°C)	36-37.5	<35 or >38.5
Urine output (ml/hour)	40-100	<20

If any measured value lies outside the normal ranges given above, or there is any doubt, seek medical advice immediately. If the patient looks unwell, they probably are.

Examining body systems

This should be done in a methodical manner, moving through each body system in turn. It is common sense to start investigating the body system that appears to be experiencing the main problem. The only exception to this general rule is when major trauma or collapse has occurred. In these cases, the resuscitation and emergency assessment guidelines should be strictly followed (see pp.30–35). A guide to examining the body systems, which outlines important symptoms and signs, is included on page 35.

Monitoring

Monitoring starts when the casualty is examined and should continue until the casualty is better or has been evacuated. Routine monitoring should be carried out every hour; if the crew is very unwell, monitoring should be carried out at least every fifteen minutes. An example of a monitoring chart for vital signs is given on pp.200–201.

Testing

There are a number of simple but very effective tests that can be performed relatively easily on board which may contribute significantly to making a diagnosis and aiding treatment. Some require specific equipment, which is readily available.
- Blood sugars
- Urine analysis (dipstick)
- Pregnancy test
- Stool colour/consistency
- Sputum colour/amount
- Temperature
- Pulse oximetry
- Blood pressure
- Peak flow

Record keeping

It is of paramount importance that details of the history and examination are recorded as you go along. Facts and figures are very easily forgotten, and the medical record may well be of considerable importance for the shore medical team. An example of a medical reporting chart is included on pp.202–203.

Emergency Care: How to Save and Preserve Life

- Resuscitation – ABC
- Assessment of a Sick or Injured Crew Member
- Managing the Unconscious Crew Member
- Loss of Consciousness
- Choking
- Shock and Haemorrhage
- Chest Pain
- Allergy and Anaphylaxis
- Cold Injuries and Hypothermia
- Immersion and Drowning
- Heat Illness
- Diabetic Emergencies
- Burns

RESUSCITATION – ABC

If a crew member collapses on the boat or is recovered unconscious from the water, rapid resuscitation is vitally important and literally every second counts. The basic life support and advanced life support algorithms should be known and rehearsed by the medic and captain on a regular basis, so that they become second nature – this practice may save lives.

Basic life support

The basic life support (BLS) algorithm is very simple and gives a framework to help you think when the unthinkable happens. First, stabilize the neck (cervical spine) if there is any chance of neck injury (see pp.164–165). The algorithms prioritize the immediate life-threatening problems, so that opening and maintaining an adequate **A**irway precedes assessment and treatment of **B**reathing, which then leads on to assessment and treatment of **C**irculation (ABC).

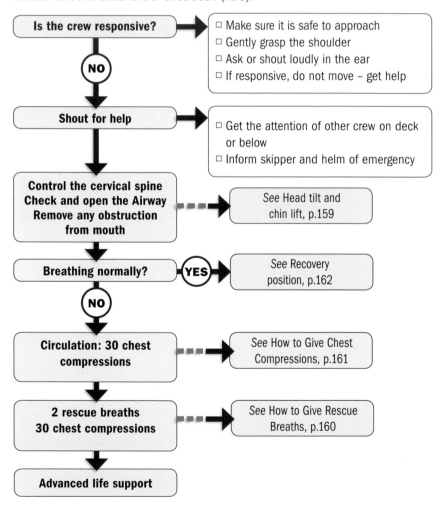

| Is the crew responsive? | | ☐ Make sure it is safe to approach
☐ Gently grasp the shoulder
☐ Ask or shout loudly in the ear
☐ If responsive, do not move – get help |

NO

| Shout for help | | ☐ Get the attention of other crew on deck or below
☐ Inform skipper and helm of emergency |

Control the cervical spine
Check and open the Airway
Remove any obstruction from mouth ----▶ See Head tilt and chin lift, p.159

Breathing normally? **YES** ▶ See Recovery position, p.162

NO

Circulation: 30 chest compressions ----▶ See How to Give Chest Compressions, p.161

2 rescue breaths
30 chest compressions ----▶ See How to Give Rescue Breaths, p.160

Advanced life support

Advanced life support

The advanced life support (ALS) algorithm is more complex, requires more skills, and assumes that there is an automated external defibrillator (AED) on board, together with adrenaline (used in resuscitation). First, stabilize the neck (cervical spine) if there is any chance of neck injury (*see* pp.164–165).

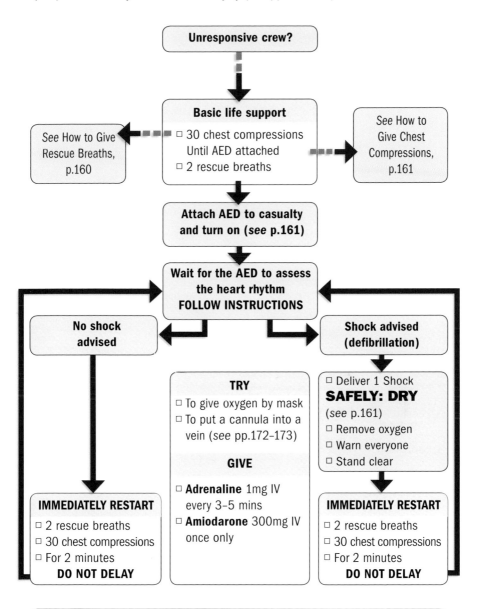

Unresponsive crew?

Basic life support
- 30 chest compressions
  Until AED attached
- 2 rescue breaths

See How to Give Rescue Breaths, p.160

See How to Give Chest Compressions, p.161

Attach AED to casualty and turn on (*see* p.161)

Wait for the AED to assess the heart rhythm FOLLOW INSTRUCTIONS

No shock advised

Shock advised (defibrillation)

TRY
- To give oxygen by mask
- To put a cannula into a vein (*see* pp.172–173)

GIVE
- **Adrenaline** 1mg IV every 3–5 mins
- **Amiodarone** 300mg IV once only

- Deliver 1 Shock
  SAFELY: DRY
  (*see* p.161)
- Remove oxygen
- Warn everyone
- Stand clear

IMMEDIATELY RESTART
- 2 rescue breaths
- 30 chest compressions
- For 2 minutes
  DO NOT DELAY

IMMEDIATELY RESTART
- 2 rescue breaths
- 30 chest compressions
- For 2 minutes
  DO NOT DELAY

Continue until the crew is breathing, or medical help arrives, or you are exhausted and cannot continue

ASSESSMENT OF A SICK OR INJURED CREW MEMBER

When faced with a severely sick or injured casualty with multiple problems, every second counts. It is important that you are able to work out rapidly what tasks to carry out and in what order. The system of primary and secondary survey is an excellent framework for organizing your actions. Like the resuscitation guidelines, the surveys should be practiced regularly by captain and medic until they become second nature.

This framework prioritizes the immediate, life-threatening problems. It is essential to deal with each stage adequately before moving on to the next. For example, the unconscious casualty will not survive for very long without an adequate Airway, which must be secured before moving on to Breathing.

THE PRIMARY SURVEY

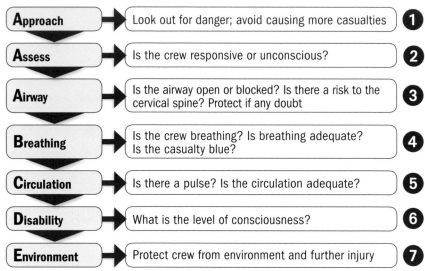

Approach → Look out for danger; avoid causing more casualties ❶

Assess → Is the crew responsive or unconscious? ❷

Airway → Is the airway open or blocked? Is there a risk to the cervical spine? Protect if any doubt ❸

Breathing → Is the crew breathing? Is breathing adequate? Is the casualty blue? ❹

Circulation → Is there a pulse? Is the circulation adequate? ❺

Disability → What is the level of consciousness? ❻

Environment → Protect crew from environment and further injury ❼

❶ Avoid self-injury while approaching injured crew

☐ Clear obstacles
☐ Avoid electrical cables, gas lines etc.
☐ Wear protective equipment
☐ Level the vessel

❷ Assessing the crew: responsive or unconscious?

Assess	Action
☐ Speak loudly in crew's ear ☐ Firmly grasp the shoulder ☐ Normal response: breathing and circulation adequate	☐ If normal response, maintain crew's comfort and go to secondary survey ☐ If abnormal response, complete primary survey

③ Airway and cervical spine protection

Assess	Action
□ Unconscious? □ Distressed? □ Seesaw chest? □ Noisy breathing? □ Effort on inspiration? □ Injury to mouth/face/neck?	□ Stabilize the cervical spine if any history of injury to head or neck (see pp.164-65) □ Open airway using "head tilt/chin lift" method (see p.159) □ Look in the mouth for obstructing objects □ Use airway device if available (see pp.159-60)

④ Breathing

Assess	Action
□ Crew blue or pale? □ Chest moving up and down? □ Rapid, shallow breathing? □ Measure rate of breathing	□ Start BLS if not breathing □ Give oxygen if breathing □ Put in the recovery position if this helps □ Treat pneumothorax if possible (see p.180)

⑤ Circulation and control of bleeding

Assess	Action
□ Confused or anxious? □ Cold, sweaty face, hands, feet? □ Obvious bleeding? □ Measure pulse rate, blood pressure, and capillary refill	□ Start BLS if no pulse □ Place crew horizontal, legs above heart □ Control bleeding (see p.70) □ Insert a cannula into a vein (see pp.172-73) □ Give IV fluids (see pp.174-75) □ Keep warm

⑥ Disability

Assess	Action

□ Level of consciousness
   A - **A**lert
   V - responds to **V**oice
   P - responds to **P**ain
   U - **U**nresponsive
 □ Are the pupils equal and responding to light?
	□ Reduced conscious level but breathing: Place in recovery position
	 □ Continue to treat other problems
	 □ **Reassess frequently**
	 □ Keep warm

⑦ Environment: protect crew during examination

Assess	Action
□ Increasingly cool and mottled skin □ Shivering □ Low temperature	□ Keep exposure time to a minimum □ Remove crew from the exposed deck as soon as possible □ Keep crew warm and dry

THE SECONDARY SURVEY

The secondary survey is a thorough, head-to-toe evaluation of the injured casualty, comprising a complete history and examination. Its purpose is to make sure no significant medical problems or injuries have been missed. A significant "**distracting injury**," such as a compound ("open") fracture of the tibia, may mean that broken ribs are missed until days later, unless all parts of the body are examined.

The history includes all the previous medical history of the patient and the most accurate account of the events that led to the accident. The history can come from a wide range of people, especially if the casualty is unconscious.

The secondary survey can only start once the life-threatening problems have been stabilized during the primary survey, which may, in itself, be a long process.

Examining someone is a very sensitive activity, but absolutely essential if the casualty is seriously injured or sick. The examination can be confined to the ankle, if only the ankle is injured, but should be comprehensive, covering the whole body (including the back) if the casualty has fallen from a height and is unconscious. Undressing (exposing) either part of, or the whole, body is necessary when examining.

The history

AMPLE is a simple memory aid that covers all the vital elements of the history.

Allergies	These are common, especially to some antibiotics, and can be life-threatening; making a bad situation worse.
Medication	What does the crew normally take? Some medications may confuse the situation, causing symptoms in their own right.
Past illnesses	Ongoing medical complaints such as diabetes may have considerable impact on the current problem. The list of medications being taken often gives a clue to past illnesses.
Last meal	Time of the last meal gives an indication whether the stomach may be full, which increases the chance of vomiting, especially if unconscious.
Events	Finding out exactly what happened, and when, gives a good idea about the possible injuries that may be expected. A fall from the spreaders will probably lead to more serious injuries than a fall into the cockpit. Try to establish:

□ **What** happened? □ **How** did it happen?
□ **Where** did it happen? □ **Why** did it happen?
□ **When** did it happen? (for future prevention)

The examination

This must be as thorough as possible, given the circumstances. Completing a comprehensive examination in the middle of the night or during a storm is not possible. However, you must remember what hasn't been done and what still remains to be done. Keep a written record, if possible.

The basis for any examination is: **Look, Feel, Listen, Move**. There is no need to undress and examine the entire body for a stubbed toe, but it is essential to do so if the casualty has been washed over the side and recovered unconscious. Tailor the examination using common sense, but if you are in any doubt, be more thorough. Remember a body has a front, a back, and two sides; therefore the examination is not complete until the crew is log-rolled onto the side of the body to allow the back and spine to be examined. Before you begin, check for any alert bracelets or necklaces and any operation scars. Look in the pockets for medications.

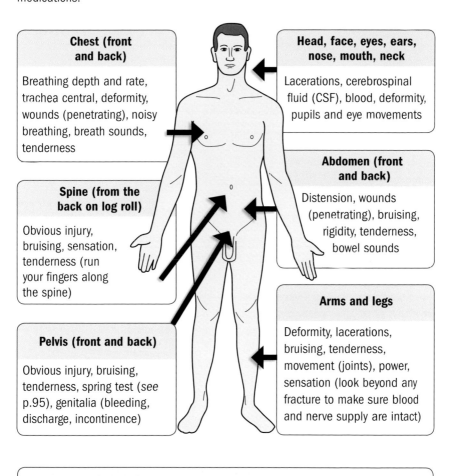

Chest (front and back)

Breathing depth and rate, trachea central, deformity, wounds (penetrating), noisy breathing, breath sounds, tenderness

Head, face, eyes, ears, nose, mouth, neck

Lacerations, cerebrospinal fluid (CSF), blood, deformity, pupils and eye movements

Spine (from the back on log roll)

Obvious injury, bruising, sensation, tenderness (run your fingers along the spine)

Abdomen (front and back)

Distension, wounds (penetrating), bruising, rigidity, tenderness, bowel sounds

Pelvis (front and back)

Obvious injury, bruising, tenderness, spring test (see p.95), genitalia (bleeding, discharge, incontinence)

Arms and legs

Deformity, lacerations, bruising, tenderness, movement (joints), power, sensation (look beyond any fracture to make sure blood and nerve supply are intact)

Remember – continue to monitor for deterioration

MANAGING THE UNCONSCIOUS CREW MEMBER

Once resuscitation, the primary survey, and the secondary survey have all been completed, you may be left with a sick or injured casualty who remains unconscious. The cause may be obvious from preceding events (such as head injury) or it may remain unclear, requiring further examination and testing that is not possible on the boat. However, even in these circumstances there are still many procedures to be carried out by the medic, captain, and crew.

The unconscious casualty is completely dependent on those around them. The objective of the entire crew is to maintain the casualty and deliver them to shore in the shortest possible time and the best possible condition. Various tasks must be undertaken to ensure the casualty does not deteriorate and has the best chance of recovery.

Maintenance of the airway
An unconscious casualty will not be able to maintain an airway when lying on his or her back.
□ Place the casualty in the recovery position (*see* below) as soon as possible.
□ Use airway devices if necessary (*see* pp.159–60)
□ Monitor the following at all times:
  – Change in colour
  – Noisy breathing
  – Chest movement
  – Rate of breathing

Recovery position
The unconscious casualty must be placed in the recovery position (*see* p.162) in order to maintain the airway and to ensure that fluids, such as vomit and saliva, drain out of the mouth and not down the airway into the lungs.
□ Use the "log roll" method of getting the patient into the recovery position if there is a chance of spinal injury (especially to the cervical spine, *see* p.163).
□ Arms and legs may need to be kept straight if they are injured or fractured.
□ Use a safe and secure position on the boat, where the unconscious casualty will not fall forwards or backwards as the boat rolls.

Injuries
□ All fractures must be splinted/immobilized if possible.
□ When bleeding has been controlled, all wounds must be cleaned thoroughly and dressed with a sterile dressing.
□ All injuries should be reviewed every few hours if there is a delay in evacuation.

Warmth

- Make sure the casualty is warm and dry.
- Monitor the temperature with a thermometer under the armpit.

Pain relief

- Paradoxically, the casualty, although unconscious, may still be affected by pain, which may be extremely severe, especially on being moved.
- Look for signs of pain (see p.111)
- Use pain relief carefully:
  - Try not to give opiates (morphine) to head-injured patients
  - If you do use opiates, monitor the rate and depth of respiration
- Use nonsedating painkillers (such as diclofenac suppositories)
- Use nerve blocks where possible (see p.185)
- Immobilize fractures and attempt to reduce the broken ends (see pp.192–95).

Pressure areas and sores

- An immobile casualty will start to develop pressure sores on the skin they are lying on if they are left in the same position for several hours. Pressure sores may also begin to develop underneath padded or inflatable splints that have been applied to fracture sites.
- Pressure sores will develop more quickly if the casualty is injured, cold, incontinent, poorly hydrated, or has low blood pressure.
- It may be necessary to log roll the casualty from side to side every few hours, depending on other injuries.
- The casualty may have been secured on a makeshift, rigid spinal board, such as a storm board, to get them down the companionway safely. They should be carefully taken off this as soon as possible.

Urinary catheter and nasogastric tube

- If the unconscious crew member is going to stay on board for more than a few hours, it is essential to put in a urinary catheter (see p.187). Full bladders are painful.
- Be careful if there is blood at the end of the penis or coming out of the vagina.
- A nasogastric tube (see p.186) is also very useful for two reasons:
  - To empty the stomach of food, to avoid vomiting
  - As a way of keeping the person hydrated
- Do not insert a nasogastric tube if the casualty may have a head injury. Use the mouth instead if accessible.

Hydration

It is imperative to make sure the casualty receives adequate fluid while unconscious, but it is very difficult to assess exactly how much fluid should be given. As a general guide, 3L a day should be sufficient for a person weighing 70kg. However, this amount may need to be altered depending on:
- Blood loss due to either external or internal injuries

- Fluid loss from sweating, in a hot climate
- Burn injuries (*see* pp.60–63)
- Blood pressure: low blood pressure may be increased by giving additional fluid in 250ml amounts intravenously

There are various ways of administering fluid and judging the adequacy of hydration (*see* pp.70–73).

Easy tests on board

Some tests are easy to perform on board the boat, and may give very useful information.
- Blood sugar with testing sticks (essential in diabetics)
- Urine with testing sticks (for blood, sugar, signs of kidney or bladder damage)
- Pregnancy testing kit
- Pulse oximetry

Monitoring vital signs

Monitoring is an essential task in order to spot and correct deterioration at an early stage. Make sure you use a record chart (*see* pp.204–205), and note down the following values every hour as a minimum:
- Pulse
- Blood pressure
- Respiratory rate
- Urine output (if possible)
- Temperature
- Pupil reactions
- Conscious state AVPU: Alert; Vocal stimuli provoke response; Painful stimuli provoke response; Unresponsive (*see* p.168)/Glasgow Coma Score (*see* p.169)

Communication and evacuation

- Seek medical advice early
- Communicate effectively: Prioritize information
- Identify the person you are speaking with
- Evacuate at the first opportunity
- Do not minimize the seriousness of the situation to shore
- Make sure you know how to evacuate a casualty (*see* p.214)
- Make sure documentation goes with the casualty

LOSS OF CONSCIOUSNESS

A reduction in consciousness to the point of being unresponsive is a dramatic event with a variety of possible causes, some obvious, others not. The immediate treatment priorities are airway, breathing, and circulation (ABC). Often, the casualty is not completely unconscious but somewhat responsive.

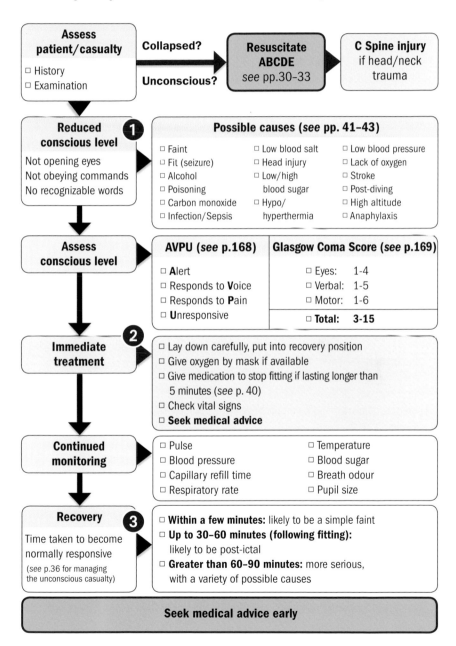

Assess patient/casualty
- History
- Examination

Collapsed?

Unconscious?

Resuscitate ABCDE *see pp.30–33*

C Spine injury if head/neck trauma

Reduced conscious level ❶
Not opening eyes
Not obeying commands
No recognizable words

Possible causes (see pp. 41–43)
- Faint
- Fit (seizure)
- Alcohol
- Poisoning
- Carbon monoxide
- Infection/Sepsis
- Low blood salt
- Head injury
- Low/high blood sugar
- Hypo/hyperthermia
- Low blood pressure
- Lack of oxygen
- Stroke
- Post-diving
- High altitude
- Anaphylaxis

Assess conscious level

AVPU (see p.168)
- **A**lert
- Responds to **V**oice
- Responds to **P**ain
- **U**nresponsive

Glasgow Coma Score (see p.169)
- Eyes: 1-4
- Verbal: 1-5
- Motor: 1-6
- **Total: 3-15**

Immediate treatment ❷
- Lay down carefully, put into recovery position
- Give oxygen by mask if available
- Give medication to stop fitting if lasting longer than 5 minutes (see p. 40)
- Check vital signs
- **Seek medical advice**

Continued monitoring
- Pulse
- Blood pressure
- Capillary refill time
- Respiratory rate
- Temperature
- Blood sugar
- Breath odour
- Pupil size

Recovery ❸
Time taken to become normally responsive
(see p.36 for managing the unconscious casualty)
- **Within a few minutes:** likely to be a simple faint
- **Up to 30–60 minutes (following fitting):** likely to be post-ictal
- **Greater than 60–90 minutes:** more serious, with a variety of possible causes

Seek medical advice early

① Assessing the casualty

A quick examination of the casualty will reveal details that may enable diagnosis. Look for:

- Vital signs (pulse, blood pressure)
- Obvious fitting
- Pupil size
- Smell of alcohol, ketones (sweet breath)
- Paralysis of one side of the face or body
- Head injury
- Any other injury and bleeding
- Rolling eye movements
- Tongue biting
- Incontinence of urine or faeces

When determining the level of consciousness, use a gradual increase in stimulation to get the casualty to respond. Start by asking for a verbal response ("Are you okay?") in a loud voice. If no response, try gripping their shoulder and gently shaking it (watch the cervical spine). If there is still no response, try a painful stimulus:

- Rub the edge of the eye socket under the eyebrow
- Rub the centre of the chest firmly
- Press a pen onto the base of a finger nail.

Try the painful stimulus on yourself first, to make sure the stimulus is reasonable and not causing lasting discomfort or injury.

② Treatment of prolonged fitting

A fit or series of fits without regaining consciousness, lasting longer than 5–10 minutes, should be treated, to avoid the risk of permanent brain damage. An episode of fitting lasting longer than 30 minutes is known as status epilepticus, and is a serious emergency that could result in permanent brain damage or death.

First line treatment – ABC and oxygen followed by:

- Diazepam 10mg
    - Use the injection form rather than the suppository (absorption is faster)
    - Repeat at 15-minute intervals up to 40mg

OR

- Lorazepam 2–4mg intravenously
    - Repeat once after 20 minutes
    - Lasts for up to 12 hours

Important: Both diazepam and lorazepam have similar actions, and they should not be used together unless under medical direction. They will sedate the casualty and reduce consciousness level, and may even stop the breathing, so use carefully. Flumazenil is an antidote, but use it under medical direction only (see pp.210–213).

③ Recovery of consciousness

The time it takes for the casualty to recover consciousness gives a guide to the possible, or even probable, diagnosis. However, the guides in terms of time are only approximate, and should not definitely exclude another diagnosis.

The post-ictal period is the phase when the casualty has stopped fitting but has not yet regained consciousness. It usually lasts less than 30 minutes, but may last several hours. The post-ictal period tends to be longer with more prolonged, generalized fitting and when more medication has been used to terminate the fit.

Causes of loss of consciousness

Fainting

Simple fainting is not uncommon and is usually caused by a temporary drop in blood pressure causing a "blackout". Precipitating factors include severe pain, panic attacks, emotional or physical shock (such as the sight of blood), and excessive heat. Sometimes the patient may twitch while unconscious, but this does not necessarily indicate epilepsy. The patient should be put in the recovery position, which helps to restore blood flow to the brain. Recovery should follow within a couple of minutes. Check for injuries if the casualty collapsed.

Fitting

There are many possible causes of fitting:

- Epilepsy
- Alcohol withdrawal
- Recreational drug withdrawal
- Strokes
- Low blood salt (hyponatraemia)
- Head injury
- Low blood sugar
- Infection
- Hyperthermia (fever in children)
- Post-diving

Fitting may be generalized, when the whole body shakes, or may be partial, when only part of the body is involved (such as the eyes or a single muscle group). These "partial" fits may be difficult to recognize as fits, but should be treated the same. Seasickness (reducing absorption of anti-epilepsy tablets), work stress, poor nutrition, and dehydration may all cause fits in known epileptics who were previously well-controlled. Epileptics sometimes get an "aura" (a feeling they are going to have a fit). It is important to get them to a safe place prior to the onset of fitting. The priority in all cases is resuscitation, followed by treatment to stop the fitting if it continues beyond 5 minutes. Checking of vital signs, particularly blood sugar, is crucial and may guide immediate treatment.

Alcohol

This is a common reason for being unrousable, but hopefully not on a boat. Fitting may occur after exceptional alcohol consumption or in heavy drinkers who are then on a dry boat. Withdrawal effects such as fitting tend to occur after 2–3 days without alcohol. A history of heavy drinking in the immediate past and breath smelling heavily of alcohol are guides to diagnosis. These casualties are at risk of vomiting and vomit entering the lungs when they are unconscious. They should be placed in the recovery position. Any prolonged fitting should be treated and carefully monitored (see p.40).

Poisoning

Poisoning may be accidental or deliberate. Any poisoning event that leads to unconsciousness is life-threatening. Prescription drugs such as antidepressants, sedatives, and heart treatment drugs may cause loss of consciousness and possibly fitting as well. If these drugs are on the boat, keep them in a safe place. Poisoning by gas is a real threat on a boat. Make sure you are not overcome when entering a cabin to rescue a casualty (see p.154 for specific treatments).

Carbon monoxide (CO)

Inhalation of carbon monoxide is a form of poisoning and is a distinct possibility on a boat that has a defective gas cooker or generator. The symptoms of this condition tend to be vague: nausea, vomiting, confusion, chest pain, and, in severe cases, eventual unconsciousness. The casualty may appear very red-faced, the colour often being described as "cherry red". If several crew members have the same symptoms, carbon monoxide poisoning should be considered. The casualty should be removed from the source and be given as much oxygen as possible if available (*see* p.154).

Infection

Loss of consciousness (LoC) and fitting may occur due to infection of the membrane covering the brain (meningitis) or infection of the brain itself (encephalitis). A history of feeling increasingly unwell (for anything from several hours to days beforehand), together with a high temperature and possibly a nonblanching rash, raises the possibility of infection. Any fitting should be treated, and high-dose antibiotics should be given intravenously as soon as possible (*see* pp.142–143 for further treatment).

Low blood salt

A low level of sodium in the blood is a condition known as hyponatraemia. The most likely reason for this is that the crew has been using only water to rehydrate, rather than rehydration salts, in warm, humid conditions, when the work rate may be high. Prevention is essential, paying attention to adequate, appropriate fluid intake. Making a firm diagnosis of hyponatraemia on a boat is impossible and would be based on suspicion only. The only treatment possible on a boat (after appropriate resuscitation has been given) would be to give rectal rehydration fluid or IV normal saline solution (*see* pp.170–171).

Head injury

Head injury sufficient to cause a period of loss of consciousness may well be associated with injuries to the spine, including the neck. Bear this in mind, and protect the cervical spine at all times. A GCS of 13 or more indicates mild injury, while a GCS of 8 or less indicates severe injury. The longer the period of LoC, the more severe the injury, and a period of LoC longer than 5 minutes should be taken very seriously. Treatment comprises resuscitation and management of the unconscious casualty (*see* pp.36–38). Any casualty who has suffered LoC due to head injury should be monitored closely for at least 24 hours following the event, because deterioration is a real possibility (*see* p.74 for further treatment).

Low/high blood sugar

High or low blood sugar may occur in known diabetics, but there are other causes of these conditions, which may lead to fitting, as well as LoC, particularly in the case of low blood sugar levels. It is imperative that you check the crew's blood sugar level as soon as possible, particularly if he or she is a known diabetic (*see* p.59 for further treatment).

Hypo/hyperthermia

Fitting and LoC are more likely with hyperthermia at body core temperatures above 40°C, whereas hypothermia is likely to cause LoC below 32°C. Treatment comprises treating the fitting initially, then reversing the hypo- or hyperthermia (for hypothermia see pp.52–53 and for hyperthermia see pp.56–57).

Low blood pressure

A systolic blood pressure lower than 70mmHg is likely to cause a reduction in conscious level. Some crew may be more susceptible to low blood pressure than others, particularly those with a history of high blood pressure or diabetes. Restoring blood flow to the head by lying the casualty down and raising the legs is the quickest treatment. Treat the cause of low blood pressure (such as blood loss) immediately, with IV access and fluid resuscitation. A heart attack may cause low blood pressure (or even a cardiac arrest in extreme cases). **Seek medical advice urgently**, as the casualty may deteriorate rapidly.

Lack of oxygen

The main reasons for lack of oxygen delivery to the brain are loss of airway and lack of effective breathing (and lack of adequate circulation, as above). LoC and possible fitting due to lack of oxygen are extremely serious and very likely to cause permanent damage. Immediate resuscitation is imperative (see p.30), and oxygen by mask should be given if possible. Fitting should be treated if it persists for longer than 5 minutes.

Stroke

A stroke is caused by lack of blood flow to part of the brain, either because of a blood clot or because of a bleed into the brain itself. LoC would be caused by a very large stroke or a smaller stroke in a critical area of the brain. Fitting may occur, as well as paralysis or abnormal movements down one side of the body. Immediate resuscitation is important, in order to restore blood and oxygen supply to the brain and limit further damage (see p.117 for further treatment).

Post-diving

A casualty who becomes unconscious soon after returning from diving is very likely to have suffered an air embolism (decompression illness). Immediate resuscitation is imperative. The patient should be placed in the recovery position if he or she is breathing and has a pulse. Oxygen should be given if available, and IV fluids administered if possible. **Seek medical advice immediately**, with a view to immediate evacuation, ideally to a decompression facility.

CHOKING

Breathing difficulty caused by choking may progress rapidly to collapse if the cause isn't promptly recognized and treatment started. This is an emergency and must be treated as such.

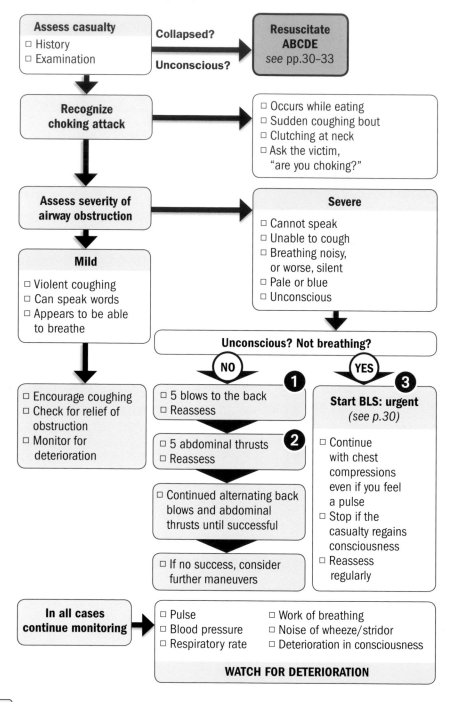

Assess casualty
- □ History
- □ Examination

Collapsed?

Unconscious?

Resuscitate ABCDE
see pp.30–33

Recognize choking attack
- □ Occurs while eating
- □ Sudden coughing bout
- □ Clutching at neck
- □ Ask the victim, "are you choking?"

Assess severity of airway obstruction

Severe
- □ Cannot speak
- □ Unable to cough
- □ Breathing noisy, or worse, silent
- □ Pale or blue
- □ Unconscious

Mild
- □ Violent coughing
- □ Can speak words
- □ Appears to be able to breathe

Unconscious? Not breathing?

NO

YES

- □ Encourage coughing
- □ Check for relief of obstruction
- □ Monitor for deterioration

1
- □ 5 blows to the back
- □ Reassess

2
- □ 5 abdominal thrusts
- □ Reassess

- □ Continued alternating back blows and abdominal thrusts until successful

- □ If no success, consider further maneuvers

3
Start BLS: urgent
(see p.30)
- □ Continue with chest compressions even if you feel a pulse
- □ Stop if the casualty regains consciousness
- □ Reassess regularly

In all cases continue monitoring
- □ Pulse
- □ Blood pressure
- □ Respiratory rate
- □ Work of breathing
- □ Noise of wheeze/stridor
- □ Deterioration in consciousness

WATCH FOR DETERIORATION

① Giving back blows

The victim must be conscious and be able to stand up for you to perform this procedure. Make sure you explain briefly what you are about to do, as a back blow may be painful.

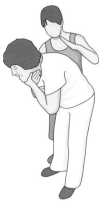

- ☐ Stand to one side, lean the crew forwards over your left arm, supporting the chest. Lean his or her upper body well forwards so that any dislodged object is more likely be expelled from the mouth.
- ☐ Give five sharp and very firm blows between the shoulder blades with the heel of your hand.
- ☐ Reassess briefly between each blow; if the object is dislodged or comes out, stop delivering blows.

Give five firm blows between the shoulder blades.

② Giving abdominal thrusts

Again, the victim must be conscious and able to stand up. Explain what you are about to do. Abdominal thrusts may be more painful than back blows.

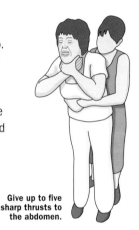

- ☐ Lean the crew member forwards from behind. Place one clenched fist in the upper abdomen, just below the ribs in the centre line. Cover it with your other hand and maintain a firm hold.
- ☐ Give up to five sharp thrusts to the abdomen.
- ☐ Reassess briefly between the thrusts, and stop if the object is dislodged or comes out.

Give up to five sharp thrusts to the abdomen.

③ Basic life support with chest compressions

If the casualty becomes unconscious, basic life support is then required. It is probably worthwhile continuing chest compressions, even if you can feel a pulse, because the chest compressions may raise the pressure in the lungs and force the object out of the airway. Continue with chest compressions until one of the following occurs:

- ☐ The object is dislodged
- ☐ There is a pulse
- ☐ Help arrives
- ☐ You are exhausted and cannot continue

④ Further treatment

Once the object is successfully dislodged, the crew member may remain wheezy and continue to have difficulty with their breathing (*see* pp.158–159 for further supportive treatment).

SHOCK AND HAEMORRHAGE

If a casualty is haemorrhaging and the bleeding is not stopped, shock may develop, which can be life-threatening. Shock occurs when there is not enough blood reaching the vital organs. Immediate action is crucial. Internal bleeding is more difficult to assess and stop. Causes of internal bleeding include penetrating injury to chest or abdomen; arm and leg bone fractures; pelvic fractures; and blunt trauma to chest or abdomen. The stomach, intestines, and uterus are also prone to internal bleeding.

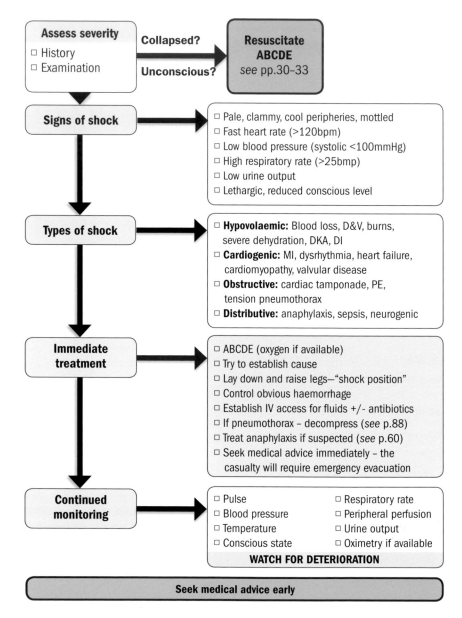

Assess severity
- History
- Examination

Collapsed?
Unconscious?

Resuscitate ABCDE see pp.30–33

Signs of shock
- Pale, clammy, cool peripheries, mottled
- Fast heart rate (>120bpm)
- Low blood pressure (systolic <100mmHg)
- High respiratory rate (>25bmp)
- Low urine output
- Lethargic, reduced conscious level

Types of shock
- **Hypovolaemic:** Blood loss, D&V, burns, severe dehydration, DKA, DI
- **Cardiogenic:** MI, dysrhythmia, heart failure, cardiomyopathy, valvular disease
- **Obstructive:** cardiac tamponade, PE, tension pneumothorax
- **Distributive:** anaphylaxis, sepsis, neurogenic

Immediate treatment
- ABCDE (oxygen if available)
- Try to establish cause
- Lay down and raise legs—"shock position"
- Control obvious haemorrhage
- Establish IV access for fluids +/- antibiotics
- If pneumothorax – decompress (see p.88)
- Treat anaphylaxis if suspected (see p.60)
- Seek medical advice immediately – the casualty will require emergency evacuation

Continued monitoring
- Pulse
- Blood pressure
- Temperature
- Conscious state
- Respiratory rate
- Peripheral perfusion
- Urine output
- Oximetry if available

WATCH FOR DETERIORATION

Seek medical advice early

IMMEDIATE TREATMENT

- ☐ Resuscitate ABCDE (*see* pp.30–33)
- ☐ Lie the casualty down and raise the legs
- ☐ Get venous access if you can and give IV fluid (*see* p.172).

How to stop bleeding

Direct pressure
- ☐ Wearing gloves, apply very firm pressure.
- ☐ Press on either side if there are bones sticking out.
- ☐ Continue for as long as possible or until the bleeding stops.

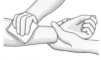

Apply direct pressure.

Tourniquet
Use in extreme circumstances only, as this procedure may dangerously reduce blood flow to distal arm or leg. A tourniquet is essential to stop major haemorrhage following traumatic limb amputation.

Tie a tourniquet.

Splinting/Immobilization
Put the broken ends of the bones back as close as possible to the normal position. Splint firmly (not too tightly) in position. If the pelvis is fractured, hold it together with a strap or sling. Keep casualty as still as possible in a bunk until evacuated.

Elevation
Elevating the injured part of the body, usually an arm or leg, will reduce bleeding from veins and skin, but is unlikely to be effective with arterial bleeding.

Haemostatic dressing/powder
Apply to wound, either as a gauze pack or powder. This must be used with direct pressure, not alone.

Tranexamic acid
Used either as an IV injection or tablet. Must be used under direct medical advice.

Young and older casualties
Younger people compensate for blood loss to a much greater extent than older people, so older people should be treated sooner. Conversely, young people starting to show symptoms of blood loss are in serious trouble and need urgent treatment.

Blood loss in fractures
- ☐ Fractured humerus, up to 500ml
- ☐ Fractured femur, over 1,000ml per leg
- ☐ Fractured pelvis, 2,000ml or more

Medications that may complicate blood loss
- ☐ Blood-thinning drugs such as aspirin and warfarin are often used to treat heart conditions. They make bleeding much worse and should be stopped.
- ☐ Beta blockers, such as atenolol, slow the heart rate and may hide or suppress the rapid-pulse response to significant blood loss.
- ☐ Antiseasickness tablets may sometimes cause drowsiness, reducing the conscious state in the event of blood loss.

CHEST PAIN

The heart is basically a muscle and depends on its blood supply to keep going. If the blood supply is reduced, this may cause pain (angina). If the supply reduces even further, this can cause a heart attack (myocardial infarction), which is usually extremely painful.

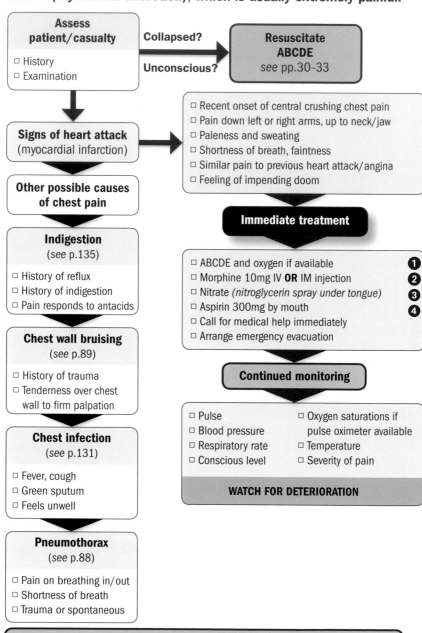

Assess patient/casualty
- History
- Examination

Collapsed?
Unconscious?

Resuscitate ABCDE
see pp.30–33

Signs of heart attack (myocardial infarction)

- Recent onset of central crushing chest pain
- Pain down left or right arms, up to neck/jaw
- Paleness and sweating
- Shortness of breath, faintness
- Similar pain to previous heart attack/angina
- Feeling of impending doom

Other possible causes of chest pain

Immediate treatment

Indigestion (see p.135)
- History of reflux
- History of indigestion
- Pain responds to antacids

- ABCDE and oxygen if available ❶
- Morphine 10mg IV **OR** IM injection ❷
- Nitrate *(nitroglycerin spray under tongue)* ❸
- Aspirin 300mg by mouth ❹
- Call for medical help immediately
- Arrange emergency evacuation

Chest wall bruising (see p.89)
- History of trauma
- Tenderness over chest wall to firm palpation

Continued monitoring

Chest infection (see p.131)
- Fever, cough
- Green sputum
- Feels unwell

- Pulse
- Blood pressure
- Respiratory rate
- Conscious level
- Oxygen saturations if pulse oximeter available
- Temperature
- Severity of pain

WATCH FOR DETERIORATION

Pneumothorax (see p.88)
- Pain on breathing in/out
- Shortness of breath
- Trauma or spontaneous

Seek medical advice early

TREATMENT OF HEART ATTACKS

If the casualty collapses, rapid resuscitation and advanced life support are imperative. The cause of collapse may be an irregular heart rhythm (ventricular fibrillation or tachycardia), which stops the heart pumping blood properly. Rapid defibrillation with an AED may return the heart back to normal rhythm. In less serious heart attacks, there are a few simple treatments that may reduce the chance of the heart attack getting worse or happening again – morphine, oxygen, nitrate spray, and aspirin (MONA):

❶ Oxygen by face mask (if available)

Place the mask on the casualty's face as soon as possible, with a flow rate of 5-10L per minute. This will increase the supply of oxygen to the heart, reducing further damage to the heart muscle.

❷ Morphine 10mg intramuscular injection

Give this injection into the shoulder, firmly (see p.175). Give an injection of anti-nausea medicine (cyclizine) as well. This will reduce the levels of pain and anxiety in the casualty and lessen the strain on the heart.

❸ Nitrate spray under the tongue

Give a glyceryl trinitrate spray twice under the tongue as soon as possible. The spray will dilate the arteries supplying the heart, increasing the blood supply. If the chest pain does not go away or comes back, you can repeat the treatment. However, glyceryl trinitrate may lower the blood pressure or cause a headache if overused.

❹ Aspirin 300mg by mouth

Give in the dispersible form if possible; absorption from the stomach will be faster. Aspirin will thin the blood and reduce the chance of a clot in the arteries supplying the heart muscle.

Ongoing treatment

This depends on the physical state of the casualty. It is essential to seek medical advice straight away. If advice is not immediately available, continue treatment as follows until help is reached:
- Aspirin 150mg per day (as long as stomach is not upset/bleeding)
- Glyceryl trinitrate spray if the chest pain returns
- Morphine 5mg injections if the chest pain returns, depending on the conscious state of the casualty.

Crew with known heart problems

Any crew member with a known history of heart problems should be carefully assessed before getting on the boat (see pp.24-27). Someone who complains of chest pain while not exerting him- or herself, or who complains of worsening chest pains and reduced ability to perform routine tasks, should not get on the boat and should visit a doctor immediately.

ALLERGY AND ANAPHYLAXIS

Anaphylaxis, or anaphylactic shock, is an extreme form of allergic reaction that affects the whole body. The mouth and throat may swell, and the casualty may collapse due to low blood pressure (BP) and inability to breathe. Crew who have had anaphylactic reactions before should carry a preprepared adrenaline syringe.

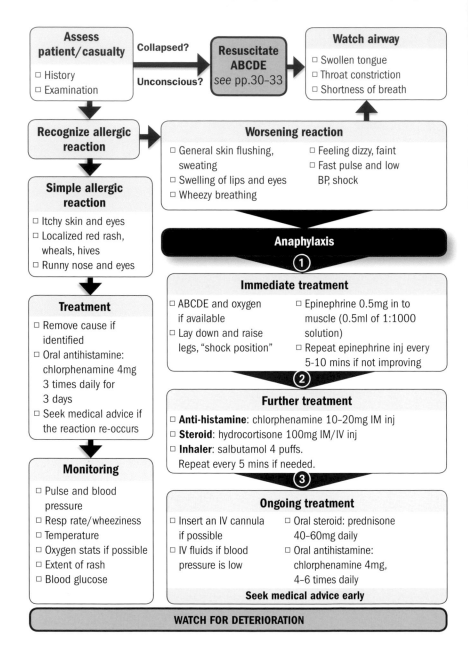

Assess patient/casualty
- □ History
- □ Examination

Collapsed?

Unconscious?

Resuscitate ABCDE
see pp.30–33

Watch airway
- □ Swollen tongue
- □ Throat constriction
- □ Shortness of breath

Recognize allergic reaction

Worsening reaction
- □ General skin flushing, sweating
- □ Swelling of lips and eyes
- □ Wheezy breathing
- □ Feeling dizzy, faint
- □ Fast pulse and low BP, shock

Simple allergic reaction
- □ Itchy skin and eyes
- □ Localized red rash, wheals, hives
- □ Runny nose and eyes

Anaphylaxis
①

Treatment
- □ Remove cause if identified
- □ Oral antihistamine: chlorphenamine 4mg 3 times daily for 3 days
- □ Seek medical advice if the reaction re-occurs

Immediate treatment
- □ ABCDE and oxygen if available
- □ Lay down and raise legs, "shock position"
- □ Epinephrine 0.5mg in to muscle (0.5ml of 1:1000 solution)
- □ Repeat epinephrine inj every 5-10 mins if not improving

②

Further treatment
- □ **Anti-histamine**: chlorphenamine 10–20mg IM inj
- □ **Steroid**: hydrocortisone 100mg IM/IV inj
- □ **Inhaler**: salbutamol 4 puffs. Repeat every 5 mins if needed.

③

Monitoring
- □ Pulse and blood pressure
- □ Resp rate/wheeziness
- □ Temperature
- □ Oxygen stats if possible
- □ Extent of rash
- □ Blood glucose

Ongoing treatment
- □ Insert an IV cannula if possible
- □ IV fluids if blood pressure is low
- □ Oral steroid: prednisone 40-60mg daily
- □ Oral antihistamine: chlorphenamine 4mg, 4-6 times daily

Seek medical advice early

WATCH FOR DETERIORATION

❶ Immediate treatment

☐ Remove the cause if possible.

☐ Lie the casualty down in a comfortable position and put the legs up.

☐ Give oxygen by face mask (5L per minute) if available.

☐ Adrenaline is the single most important treatment to stop things getting worse.

☐ Adrenaline injection 0.5mg (0.5ml of 1:1000 solution) into the front of the thigh or shoulder. This may be repeated every 5–10 minutes if the casualty is not improving. Use a different limb to inject repeat doses.

☐ Use pre-filled syringes of adrenaline if available.

☐ Adrenaline may make the pulse go faster, and increase the blood pressure. Be careful the injection doesn't go directly into a blood vessel (*see* p.175).

❷ Further treatment

The aim of the following additional treatments is to damp down the anaphylactic reaction more permanently than adrenaline is able to do and to prevent the process from starting up again.

Antihistamine injection: Chlorphenamine injection 10-20mg into the front of the thigh or shoulder.
Use a different limb to the one used for adrenaline.
Give up to 40mg per day.
Continue for 24–48 hours post reaction.

Steroid injection: Hydrocortisone 100mg IM or IV if access available.
Begins to work over several hours and has a prolonged effect.
Give up to 100mg 3 times per day.
Continue for 24–48 hours post reaction.

Inhaler: Salbutamol inhaler 4 puffs, repeated as necessary every 5 minutes.
Treats wheeze which may develop with anaphylaxis.
Continue for as long as the wheeze is present.

❸ Ongoing treatment

The goal here is to stabilize the casualty, prevent the anaphylactic reaction returning, and to secure medical help as soon as possible.

IV fluid: Fluid resuscitation may be required in the early stages if the blood pressure remains dangerously low despite the other treatments (*see* pp.172–173).

Oral steroids: Continue oral prednisolone 40-60mg per day according to symptoms.

Oral antihistamines: Continue oral chlorphenamine 4mg 3–6 times per day according to symptoms.

**Continue oral treatment until casualty is under medical care
Seek medical advice early**

COLD INJURIES AND HYPOTHERMIA

Crew who sail in cold regions are constantly exposed to freezing or near-freezing conditions, made worse by incessant wind over the deck. It is obvious that immersion in cold water is likely to cause acute hypothermia, but less obvious that prolonged exposure to wet, cold conditions on deck may cause both localized cold injury and slower onset hypothermia. Prevention is fundamental, but if symptoms are recognized, they should not be ignored; early treatment will limit injury and minimize complications.

Cold injury

Cold injury may occur after only a few minutes of exposure. Conditions just above 0°C may cause non-freezing injuries, whereas conditions below 0°C are more likely to cause freezing injury.

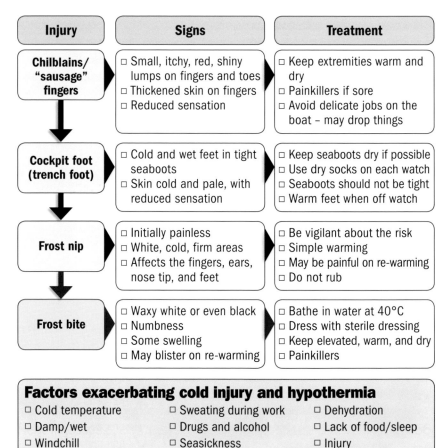

Injury	Signs	Treatment
Chilblains/ "sausage" fingers	□ Small, itchy, red, shiny lumps on fingers and toes □ Thickened skin on fingers □ Reduced sensation	□ Keep extremities warm and dry □ Painkillers if sore □ Avoid delicate jobs on the boat – may drop things
Cockpit foot (trench foot)	□ Cold and wet feet in tight seaboots □ Skin cold and pale, with reduced sensation	□ Keep seaboots dry if possible □ Use dry socks on each watch □ Seaboots should not be tight □ Warm feet when off watch
Frost nip	□ Initially painless □ White, cold, firm areas □ Affects the fingers, ears, nose tip, and feet	□ Be vigilant about the risk □ Simple warming □ May be painful on re-warming □ Do not rub
Frost bite	□ Waxy white or even black □ Numbness □ Some swelling □ May blister on re-warming	□ Bathe in water at 40°C □ Dress with sterile dressing □ Keep elevated, warm, and dry □ Painkillers

Factors exacerbating cold injury and hypothermia

□ Cold temperature   □ Sweating during work   □ Dehydration
□ Damp/wet   □ Drugs and alcohol   □ Lack of food/sleep
□ Windchill   □ Seasickness   □ Injury

Hypothermia

The onset of hypothermia may be insidious and may not be noticed until the body core temperature has dropped significantly – the crew may be lethargic, confused, and withdrawn. This state is extremely dangerous and may lead to accidents.

Prevention, early recognition, and swift action are required to avoid complications.

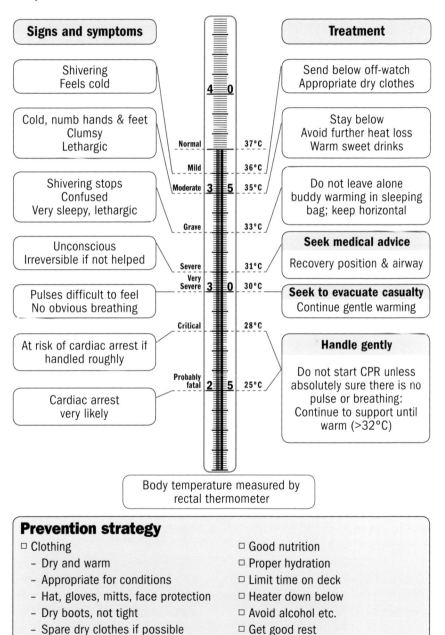

Signs and symptoms

Shivering
Feels cold

Cold, numb hands & feet
Clumsy
Lethargic

Shivering stops
Confused
Very sleepy, lethargic

Unconscious
Irreversible if not helped

Pulses difficult to feel
No obvious breathing

At risk of cardiac arrest if handled roughly

Cardiac arrest
very likely

Treatment

Send below off-watch
Appropriate dry clothes

Stay below
Avoid further heat loss
Warm sweet drinks

Do not leave alone
buddy warming in sleeping bag; keep horizontal

Seek medical advice
Recovery position & airway

Seek to evacuate casualty
Continue gentle warming

Handle gently

Do not start CPR unless absolutely sure there is no pulse or breathing:
Continue to support until warm (>32°C)

Normal — 37°C
Mild — 36°C
Moderate — 35°C
Grave — 33°C
Severe — 31°C
Very Severe — 30°C
Critical — 28°C
Probably fatal — 25°C

4 0
3 5
3 0
2 5

Body temperature measured by rectal thermometer

Prevention strategy

☐ Clothing
  - Dry and warm
  - Appropriate for conditions
  - Hat, gloves, mitts, face protection
  - Dry boots, not tight
  - Spare dry clothes if possible

☐ Good nutrition
☐ Proper hydration
☐ Limit time on deck
☐ Heater down below
☐ Avoid alcohol etc.
☐ Get good rest

IMMERSION AND DROWNING

Cold water immersion from falling overboard is a constant risk to all those who sail in water with a temperature under 25°C (the majority of world's seas). Several physiological responses occur in the body following immersion, and the ability to cope with them will have a bearing on survival. In addition, a sudden illness (such as a heart attack) may have caused the crew to fall over the side, and the event may also have caused injury.

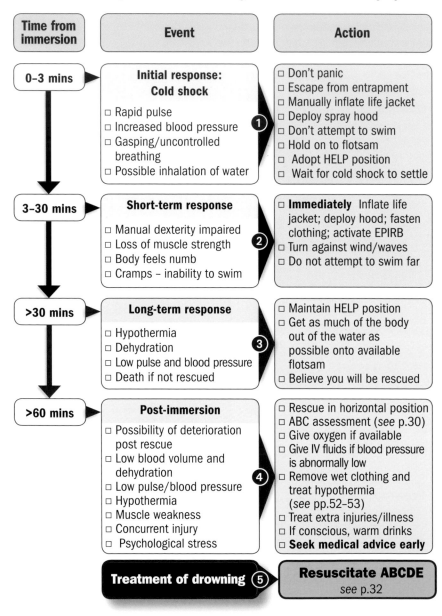

Time from immersion	Event	Action
0–3 mins	**Initial response: Cold shock** ① □ Rapid pulse □ Increased blood pressure □ Gasping/uncontrolled breathing □ Possible inhalation of water	□ Don't panic □ Escape from entrapment □ Manually inflate life jacket □ Deploy spray hood □ Don't attempt to swim □ Hold on to flotsam □ Adopt HELP position □ Wait for cold shock to settle
3–30 mins	**Short-term response** ② □ Manual dexterity impaired □ Loss of muscle strength □ Body feels numb □ Cramps – inability to swim	□ **Immediately** Inflate life jacket; deploy hood; fasten clothing; activate EPIRB □ Turn against wind/waves □ Do not attempt to swim far
>30 mins	**Long-term response** ③ □ Hypothermia □ Dehydration □ Low pulse and blood pressure □ Death if not rescued	□ Maintain HELP position □ Get as much of the body out of the water as possible onto available flotsam □ Believe you will be rescued
>60 mins	**Post-immersion** ④ □ Possibility of deterioration post rescue □ Low blood volume and dehydration □ Low pulse/blood pressure □ Hypothermia □ Muscle weakness □ Concurrent injury □ Psychological stress	□ Rescue in horizontal position □ ABC assessment (see p.30) □ Give oxygen if available □ Give IV fluids if blood pressure is abnormally low □ Remove wet clothing and treat hypothermia (see pp.52–53) □ Treat extra injuries/illness □ If conscious, warm drinks □ **Seek medical advice early**

Treatment of drowning ⑤ **Resuscitate ABCDE** *see p.32*

❶ Initial response: cold shock (0–3 minutes)

Respiration becomes rapid and gasping, and the abrupt increase in blood pressure may precipitate a heart attack or stroke in the vulnerable. Wait for the effects of sudden immersion to settle, which should happen in a few minutes. Holding onto available flotsam will have a stabilizing and reassuring effect.

❷ Short term response (3–30 minutes)

Manual dexterity will quickly become impaired, so complete all essential tasks immediately. Seawater exerts a "squeeze" on the body, causing dehydration and the possibility of circulatory collapse on being rescued. Get as much of the body onto flotsam as possible, to minimize heat loss. Maintain HELP position (Heat Escape Lessening Procedure), and bunch up close with any others.

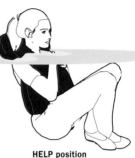

HELP position

❸ Long term response (30 minutes and longer)

The onset of hypothermia is swift, especially in colder water, and may be fatal if rescue is delayed (for treatment *see* p.53). Believe you will be rescued, but leave the rescuing to the rescuers, and do not attempt to swim any distance yourself.

❹ Post-immersion response (60 minutes and longer)

It is well known that casualties may collapse at the time of rescue or shortly afterwards (circum-rescue collapse). This is due to several factors:

☐ Loss of hydrostatic support to the lower body, causing circulatory collapse on removal from the water, exacerbated by dehydration
☐ Acute lung injury, caused by a significant amount of water entering the lungs
☐ Profound hypothermia
☐ Underlying injury or illness

The main elements of treatment are to resuscitate the casualty if unconscious (*see* p.30), treat the hypothermia (*see* p.53), and monitor pulse, blood pressure, respiration, and level of consciousness. Watch for signs of deterioration. It is vital to check for injuries. Most importantly, **seek medical advice at an early stage.**

❺ Treatment of drowning

☐ Assess ABCDE immediately (see p.32) – assess any concurrent injury or illness.
☐ Do not waste time trying to empty water from the lungs.
☐ The crew may have water in the stomach and may vomit. If vomiting occurs, turn the crew onto one side and clear the mouth of vomit to protect the airway.
☐ Treat hypothermia (*see* p.53) and keep crew as dry and warm as possible.
☐ Continue resuscitating until the casualty has a temperature greater than 32°C and is breathing, medical help arrives, or you are exhausted and cannot continue.

Acute lung injury may affect breathing over the next 24–48 hours, causing shortness of breath/fast breathing, coughing, a rapid pulse, and possible collapse. If water has entered the lungs, give oxygen and evacuate. **Seek medical advice early**.

HEAT ILLNESSES

This is often an unrecognized hazard, just as dangerous as cold injury and hypothermia. Boats that venture to the tropical regions, particularly the horse latitudes, are at risk, especially while racing, when the work rate is high. However, it is not necessary for the air temperature to be particularly high; a combination of high humidity (preventing heat loss by sweating), lack of acclimatization, high work rate, and predisposing factors may precipitate heat illness.

Illness	Symptoms/signs	Treatment
Heat Cramps Possibly due to lack of salts	□ Usually leg cramps that occur during or after exercise □ Patient may be fit and acclimatized	□ Oral rehydration with salt replacement drink □ Increase regular salt intake with food while in hot climate
Prickly heat Blocked, inflamed, infected sweat glands	□ Red, raised, itchy spots on skin usually covered by clothing (hands spared) □ May become infected:boils, spots □ Reduced sweating due to blocked sweat glands	□ Keep skin clean with good hygiene □ Keep cool, reduce work load □ Relieve itching (chlorphenamine) □ Antibiotics may be required to treat infected skin (flucloxacillin)
Heat exhaustion Water and salt loss due to sweating. Water losses may be several litres	□ Fatigue, weakness □ Heavy sweating □ Muscle cramps □ Rapid pulse □ Low blood pressure □ Rapid breathing □ Urine output less and dark in colour □ Loss of consciousness	□ Move to cool shade, lay down □ Cool with wet covers (e.g. a sheet) and fanning □ Oral rehydration with salt replacement drink - A few litres may be required - IV or rectal route if unconscious (see p.171)
Heat stroke Core temp>40°C Reduced sweating, prickly heat, not acclimatized	□ Hot, dry skin □ Headache □ Nausea, vomiting □ Weakness, staggering □ Increasing anxiety, confusion, restlessness □ Low blood sugar □ Fitting □ Loss of consciousness	□ Move to shade, lay down □ Cool with wet covers (e.g. a sheet), ice packs, fanning □ Cool IV or rectal fluids (see p.171): 1L initially. Usually not grossly dehydrated □ Measure blood sugar level and correct – often low □ **Seek medical advice**

Taking the temperature

Oral temperature readings are likely to be more accurate than those taken under the armpit. Take great care if the casualty is unconscious.

Severity of hyperthermia

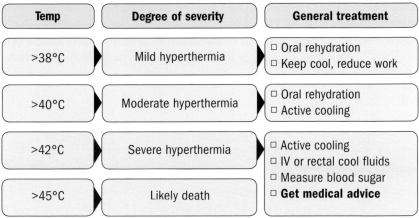

Temp	Degree of severity	General treatment
>38°C	Mild hyperthermia	☐ Oral rehydration ☐ Keep cool, reduce work
>40°C	Moderate hyperthermia	☐ Oral rehydration ☐ Active cooling
>42°C	Severe hyperthermia	☐ Active cooling ☐ IV or rectal cool fluids ☐ Measure blood sugar ☐ **Get medical advice**
>45°C	Likely death	

Factors increasing the risk of hyperthermia

Crew factors
- ☐ Dehydration (diarrhoea, menstruation)
- ☐ Diabetes
- ☐ Lack of sleep
- ☐ Reduced food intake
- ☐ Fever, infection
- ☐ Alcohol
- ☐ Old age
- ☐ Sunburn

Environmental factors
- ☐ Increased air temperature
- ☐ Increased solar heat
- ☐ Increased humidity
- ☐ Decreased wind speed

Work load
- ☐ Working at near maximum heart rate for long periods

Medication
- ☐ Atropine
- ☐ Anticholinergics
- ☐ Amphetamines
- ☐ Cocaine/ecstasy
- ☐ Antihistamines
- ☐ Beta blockers
- ☐ Diuretics
- ☐ Tricyclic antidepressants
- ☐ Prochlorperazine
- ☐ Theophylline

Prevention
- ☐ Identification of those at risk
- ☐ Team approach to rehydration
- ☐ Ready supply of rehydration drinks on deck
- ☐ Monitoring of work rate
- ☐ Early recognition of symptoms

Rehydration fluid

When a crew member is dehydrated, it is essential to replace lost salts, as well as water. Therefore, rehydrate with salt replacement drinks. If the crew is only given water on a continual basis, hyponatraemia (low sodium levels in the blood) may occur, causing fitting and unconsciousness.

DIABETIC EMERGENCIES

Crew may have one of three types of diabetes: diabetes controlled by injection of insulin a few times a day; diabetes controlled with oral diabetic tablets; or diabetes that has not been diagnosed prior to getting on the boat.

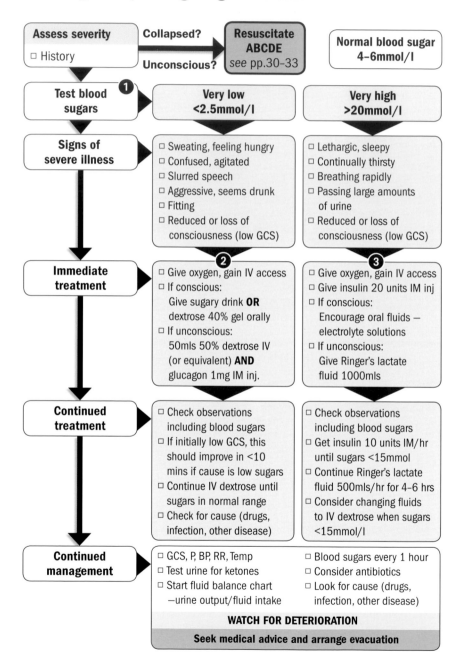

Assess severity	Collapsed?	Resuscitate ABCDE see pp.30–33		Normal blood sugar 4–6mmol/l
□ History	Unconscious?			

Test blood sugars ❶	Very low <2.5mmol/l	Very high >20mmol/l
Signs of severe illness	□ Sweating, feeling hungry □ Confused, agitated □ Slurred speech □ Aggressive, seems drunk □ Fitting □ Reduced or loss of consciousness (low GCS)	□ Lethargic, sleepy □ Continually thirsty □ Breathing rapidly □ Passing large amounts of urine □ Reduced or loss of consciousness (low GCS)
Immediate treatment	❷ □ Give oxygen, gain IV access □ If conscious: Give sugary drink **OR** dextrose 40% gel orally □ If unconscious: 50mls 50% dextrose IV (or equivalent) **AND** glucagon 1mg IM inj.	❸ □ Give oxygen, gain IV access □ Give insulin 20 units IM inj □ If conscious: Encourage oral fluids – electrolyte solutions □ If unconscious: Give Ringer's lactate fluid 1000mls
Continued treatment	□ Check observations including blood sugars □ If initially low GCS, this should improve in <10 mins if cause is low sugars □ Continue IV dextrose until sugars in normal range □ Check for cause (drugs, infection, other disease)	□ Check observations including blood sugars □ Get insulin 10 units IM/hr until sugars <15mmol □ Continue Ringer's lactate fluid 500mls/hr for 4–6 hrs □ Consider changing fluids to IV dextrose when sugars <15mmol/l
Continued management	□ GCS, P, BP, RR, Temp □ Test urine for ketones □ Start fluid balance chart —urine output/fluid intake	□ Blood sugars every 1 hour □ Consider antibiotics □ Look for cause (drugs, infection, other disease)

WATCH FOR DETERIORATION

Seek medical advice and arrange evacuation

❶ Testing blood sugar

To test the blood sugar, jab the end of a fingertip, squeeze out a drop of blood onto the testing stick, wait the required period (check the instructions) then read.

❷ Treating low blood sugar

With a known diabetic, this may be caused by excess insulin or tablets, together with lack of food or strenuous exercise. Some diabetics will know if they are having a "hypo", others may just collapse. Very low blood sugar in nondiabetics is unusual and may be due to drugs, alcohol, malaria, or an accidental dose of insulin or tablets.

Giving sugar

This can be in the form of a biscuit or sweet drink, if the casualty is conscious, or a concentrated 40% dextrose gel, placed under the tongue, rubbed in to the cheek, or swallowed. Do not put food in the casualty's mouth if he or she is unconscious. It may be aspirated into the lungs.

Glucagon

If the casualty is unconscious, consider giving glucagon 1mg intramuscularly (in to the shoulder or front of thigh), or intravenously if access is available.

History

With a known diabetic, find out when the last dose of insulin or tablet was given and the time of the last meal. Doses may need to be altered. With a casualty who is not a diabetic, find out if this has happened before and any history of drugs or illnesses.

❸ Treating high blood sugar

With a known diabetic, this may be due to too little insulin or too few tablets, or it may mean the casualty is unwell, with an infection for instance. An unknown diabetic who is having problems for the first time will need medical help as soon as possible. If there are testing sticks for urine on board, test the urine for sugar and ketones. The medical advisor will want this information. As the patient improves, the level of sugar and ketones in the urine should reduce.

Insulin

On the boat, the best way to treat is to give insulin injections intramuscularly into the shoulder or front of thigh. Give 20 units at first, then 10 units per hour until the sugar level starts to fall. Seek medical advice early to guide insulin management.

Fluid

The casualty will probably be very dehydrated. Give 1L of fluid intravenously over the first 30 minutes if you have IV fluid on board and can gain access. If IV access is not possible, use the rectal route (see p.188). After 30 minutes, lessen the amount of fluid to about 250-500ml per hour. The aim is to keep urine output at about 50-100ml per hour. Seek medical advice early to guide fluid management.

If the sugars remain too high after one hour

Medical advice is absolutely necessary at this time. It is very important to gain IV access and to pass a urinary catheter. Consider putting in a nasogastric (NG) tube to empty the stomach (particularly if the casualty is unconscious); this can be a route for giving fluid. If the casualty has a temperature above 38°C, give a dose of IV antibiotic. Check allergies first.

BURNS

Any significant burn should be recognized as a major injury affecting the whole body and assessed with primary and secondary surveys to ensure no additional injuries are overlooked (see pp.32–35). The airway may be particularly at risk, especially with fires in enclosed spaces, such as the galley. The casualty may get worse in the hours after the accident. The aim of treatment is to stop the burning process as quickly as possible, to limit damage. After immediate resuscitation, appropriate fluid treatment is absolutely crucial.

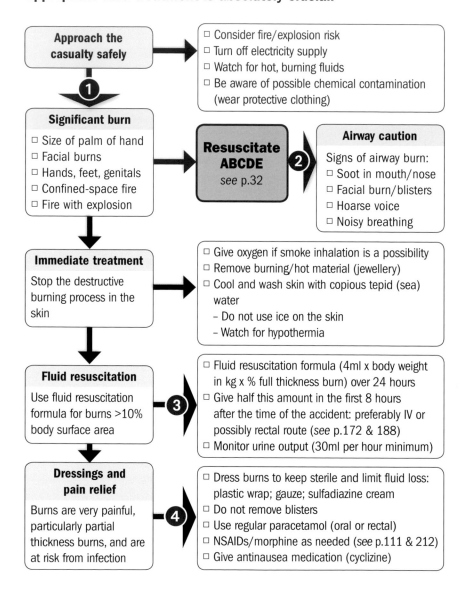

Approach the casualty safely

- ☐ Consider fire/explosion risk
- ☐ Turn off electricity supply
- ☐ Watch for hot, burning fluids
- ☐ Be aware of possible chemical contamination (wear protective clothing)

①

Significant burn

- ☐ Size of palm of hand
- ☐ Facial burns
- ☐ Hands, feet, genitals
- ☐ Confined-space fire
- ☐ Fire with explosion

Resuscitate ABCDE
see p.32

②

Airway caution

Signs of airway burn:
- ☐ Soot in mouth/nose
- ☐ Facial burn/blisters
- ☐ Hoarse voice
- ☐ Noisy breathing

Immediate treatment

Stop the destructive burning process in the skin

- ☐ Give oxygen if smoke inhalation is a possibility
- ☐ Remove burning/hot material (jewellery)
- ☐ Cool and wash skin with copious tepid (sea) water
  - – Do not use ice on the skin
  - – Watch for hypothermia

Fluid resuscitation

Use fluid resuscitation formula for burns >10% body surface area

③

- ☐ Fluid resuscitation formula (4ml x body weight in kg x % full thickness burn) over 24 hours
- ☐ Give half this amount in the first 8 hours after the time of the accident: preferably IV or possibly rectal route (see p.172 & 188)
- ☐ Monitor urine output (30ml per hour minimum)

Dressings and pain relief

Burns are very painful, particularly partial thickness burns, and are at risk from infection

④

- ☐ Dress burns to keep sterile and limit fluid loss: plastic wrap; gauze; sulfadiazine cream
- ☐ Do not remove blisters
- ☐ Use regular paracetamol (oral or rectal)
- ☐ NSAIDs/morphine as needed (see p.111 & 212)
- ☐ Give antinausea medication (cyclizine)

History

□ Finding out exactly what happened as soon as possible may give some idea as to the severity of the injury.
□ Try to find out exactly when the accident happened (it may be obvious), as this will guide fluid resuscitation.
□ Factors causing more severe burns include: prolonged exposure; falling unconscious for any period; contact with petrol; confined space; explosion.

❶ Examination: Assessment of burns

Burn area

□ The area of a burn is estimated as a percentage of the body surface area (BSA).
□ The area of full thickness burn should be estimated, as this type causes more fluid loss and more significant complications.
□ Larger burn areas cause more complications.
□ Mildly reddened skin may become obvious full thickness burn over the hours following the accident.
□ Knowing the area of full thickness burn is important, and there are various ways of estimating it.
□ For small burns, the area can be estimated by assuming the area of the casualty's palm is 1% BSA and then mapping the area of burn.
□ For larger burns, there is the "rule of nines". This assumes each region of the body is approximately 9% BSA (*see* p.62 for body map).

**The area of full thickness burn is frequently underestimated.
Keep monitoring and reassess the type and area of burn.**

Recognizing the type of burn

Superficial burn: Reddened skin, similar to sunburn. Painful and tender to touch

Partial thickness: Blistered skin, with red, healthy, soft tissue underneath the
(PT) burn blisters. Very painful and tender, as all the nerve endings are still intact

Full thickness: Pale, leathery area, burnt through to the underlying layers. May
(FT) burn be charred, involving structures like muscle, tendon, and bone. The burn itself tends not to be painful, as all the nerve endings have been destroyed. However, the area around an FT burn may be extremely painful

Significant burns

Burns to particular regions of the body are very significant because of longer term complications: face, hands, feet, genitals.

**If significant burns occur,
seek medical advice immediately.**

Rule of Nines

☐ Each region of the body (arm, front of leg, back of leg, front of chest, back of chest) counts as 9% BSA.

☐ Count obvious FT burns and blistered skin. Exclude reddened skin, but monitor, as these areas may progress to FT burn and will need adding into the total area.

❷ Risks to the airway

The airway is always at risk from significant burns. With burns of this type, you should seek medical advice immediately, but the situation could become life-threatening as tissue swelling gets worse in the hours after the accident.

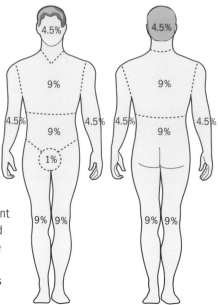

Rule of Nines: body map

Danger signs to look out for:

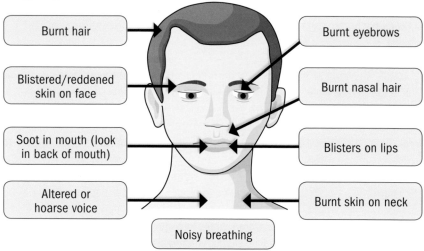

Burnt hair

Burnt eyebrows

Blistered/reddened skin on face

Burnt nasal hair

Soot in mouth (look in back of mouth)

Blisters on lips

Altered or hoarse voice

Burnt skin on neck

Noisy breathing

If any of these signs are present, seek medical advice and arrange evacuation immediately

The outlook is very grave if the casualty does begin to have difficulty breathing. The only treatment possible on a boat is to give oxygen if available. Keep the casualty sitting upright as long as possible to minimize swelling. Resuscitation should be attempted if the casualty collapses, but is unlikely to be successful. Intubation or a surgical airway should only be attempted by medical practitioners who are trained and experienced in these techniques.

❸ Fluid resuscitation

☐ Any FT or PT burn over 10% BSA may need fluid resuscitation either intravenously or rectally if unconscious.
☐ Get IV access in unburnt part as soon as possible (*see* p.172).

> **The formula for fluid resuscitation is 4ml x %BSA FT burn x weight (kgs)**
> ☐ Give half this amount in the first 8 hours following the accident.
> ☐ Give the remaining half over the next 16 hours.
> ☐ Use normal (0.9%) normal saline fluid or Ringer's lactate solution, given intravenously or rectally, or salt replacement fluid given rectally or orally.
> ☐ This is only a guide and the casualty should be reassessed frequently.

☐ Urine output:
  – A minimum 30ml per hour
  – Give a fluid bolus of 250ml if urine output is below this
  – Put in a urinary catheter if necessary
☐ Fluid resuscitation may have to continue for 36 hours or more.
☐ If you are fluid resuscitating, you must seek medical advice, to know what complications may occur and to know when to stop.

❹ Cleaning and dressing burns

☐ Burns pose risks of losing fluid from the body and infection. The dressings reduce these risks.
☐ Nonadherent material should be removed from the burn area.
☐ Chemical burns need washing with copious water – seawater if nothing else ("The solution to pollution is dilution").
☐ Replace dressings every 2–3 days according to the state of the burn.
☐ Apply silver sulfadiazine cream to burnt hands and feet and put in plastic bags.
☐ Genitals and face are often coated in petroleum jelly and not dressed.
☐ Do not remove blisters as they make excellent natural sterile dressings.
☐ Elevate affected areas as much as possible to reduce swelling.
☐ Use antibiotics if there are signs of infection (*see* p.206).

Plastic wrap If nothing else is to hand, take a few winds off a roll of plastic wrap, then use the next part for dressing. Do not wind tightly, just lay it on.
Dressing Use a paraffin-impregnated dressing with a sterile gauze patch over the top to hold it in place.
Silver sulfadiazine A cream containing sulfadiazine can be used to prevent infection and fluid loss. Do not use on the face as it may cause grey colouring of the skin.
Hydrocolloid These dressings protect wounds from contamination, hold in water, and can stay in place for a few days. They can be used for awkward areas.
Petroleum jelly To seal wounds and prevent moisture loss, petroleum jelly can be used as an emergency dressing for difficult areas, such as the face and genitals.
Honey If nothing else is available, spread honey on gauze, work it in and then use the pieces of gauze for dressing burns.

Trauma and Accidents

- Preventing Injuries
- Wounds and Bleeding
- Head Injuries
- Neck and Spinal Injuries
- Facial Injuries
- Eye Injuries
- Chest Injuries
- Abdominal Injuries
- Pelvic and Hip Injuries
- Limbs: Fracture and Dislocation
- Hand, Foot, and Ankle Injuries
- Fish Hook Injuries
- Soft Tissue Injuries
- Treating Pain

PREVENTING INJURIES

Increased risk causes increased injury, which is unwelcome on a boat because an injury to one crew member may put the rest of the crew at further risk. For example, an incapacitated crew member renders the remaining crew short-handed.

"Risk assessment" means looking at tasks on the boat with a critical eye and identifying those hazards that may result in injury if things go wrong. Once the high-risk tasks are identified, "control measures" can be used to reduce the risk of injury. A captain's briefing prior to a difficult task, such as coming alongside, should involve both of these processes. Once the hazards and risks have been identified, the crew should be assigned tasks appropriate to their level of experience.

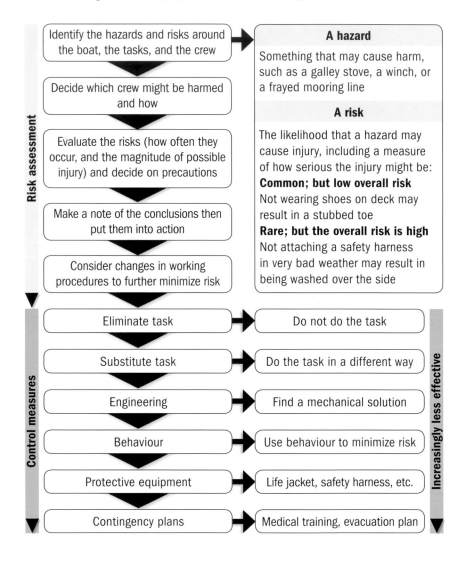

Risk assessment

- Identify the hazards and risks around the boat, the tasks, and the crew
- Decide which crew might be harmed and how
- Evaluate the risks (how often they occur, and the magnitude of possible injury) and decide on precautions
- Make a note of the conclusions then put them into action
- Consider changes in working procedures to further minimize risk

A hazard

Something that may cause harm, such as a galley stove, a winch, or a frayed mooring line

A risk

The likelihood that a hazard may cause injury, including a measure of how serious the injury might be:
Common; but low overall risk
Not wearing shoes on deck may result in a stubbed toe
Rare; but the overall risk is high
Not attaching a safety harness in very bad weather may result in being washed over the side

Control measures — **Increasingly less effective**

Eliminate task	Do not do the task
Substitute task	Do the task in a different way
Engineering	Find a mechanical solution
Behaviour	Use behaviour to minimize risk
Protective equipment	Life jacket, safety harness, etc.
Contingency plans	Medical training, evacuation plan

Risk areas of the yacht

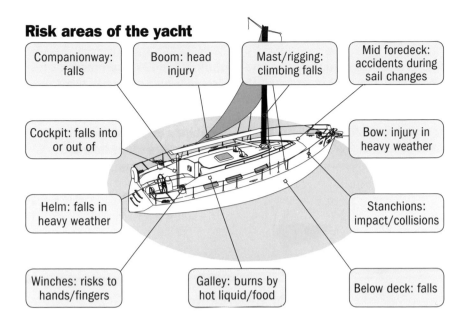

Companionway: falls

Boom: head injury

Mast/rigging: climbing falls

Mid foredeck: accidents during sail changes

Cockpit: falls into or out of

Bow: injury in heavy weather

Helm: falls in heavy weather

Winches: risks to hands/fingers

Galley: burns by hot liquid/food

Stanchions: impact/collisions

Below deck: falls

Risk areas of the crew

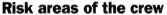
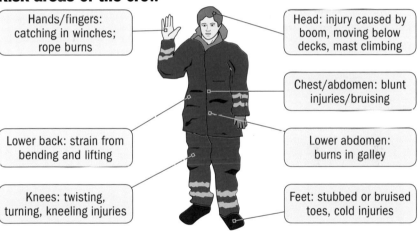

Hands/fingers: catching in winches; rope burns

Head: injury caused by boom, moving below decks, mast climbing

Chest/abdomen: blunt injuries/bruising

Lower back: strain from bending and lifting

Lower abdomen: burns in galley

Knees: twisting, turning, kneeling injuries

Feet: stubbed or bruised toes, cold injuries

Golden rules of injury prevention

□ One hand for the ship and one hand for yourself
□ Watch out for the boom (at all times)
□ Watch out below in rough weather
□ Wear something on your feet in wet areas of the boat
□ Wear your harness and clip at night and in rough weather

□ Wear sailing trousers and a galley safety strap when cooking
□ Keep fit
□ Obtain knowledge and experience
□ Consume adequate food and fluids
□ Get some sleep whenever you can
□ Avoid alcohol and drugs on board
□ Communicate

WOUNDS AND BLEEDING

Injuries that cause wounds and bleeding are very common on boats. The ability to treat them rapidly and competently is crucial and will minimize complications. Taking the correct measures to stem bleeding will prevent a drama from becoming a crisis and should be within the capability of the skipper and medic. A structured approach, and an awareness of how to prevent complications, should give the best chance of success.

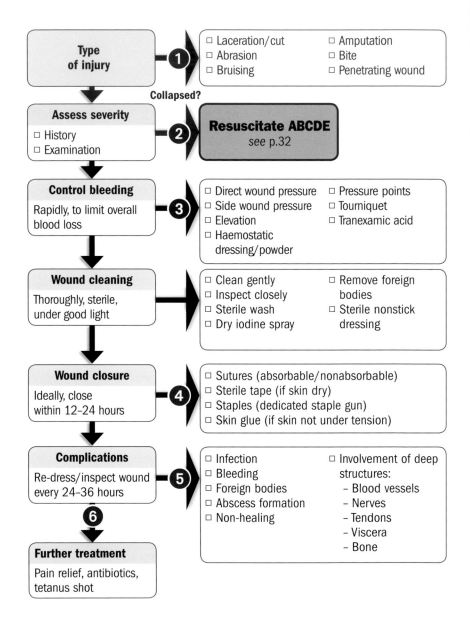

Type of injury — **1**
- □ Laceration/cut
- □ Abrasion
- □ Bruising
- □ Amputation
- □ Bite
- □ Penetrating wound

Collapsed?

Assess severity
- □ History
- □ Examination

— **2** — **Resuscitate ABCDE** *see p.32*

Control bleeding
Rapidly, to limit overall blood loss — **3**
- □ Direct wound pressure
- □ Side wound pressure
- □ Elevation
- □ Haemostatic dressing/powder
- □ Pressure points
- □ Tourniquet
- □ Tranexamic acid

Wound cleaning
Thoroughly, sterile, under good light
- □ Clean gently
- □ Inspect closely
- □ Sterile wash
- □ Dry iodine spray
- □ Remove foreign bodies
- □ Sterile nonstick dressing

Wound closure
Ideally, close within 12–24 hours — **4**
- □ Sutures (absorbable/nonabsorbable)
- □ Sterile tape (if skin dry)
- □ Staples (dedicated staple gun)
- □ Skin glue (if skin not under tension)

Complications
Re-dress/inspect wound every 24–36 hours — **5**
- □ Infection
- □ Bleeding
- □ Foreign bodies
- □ Abscess formation
- □ Non-healing
- □ Involvement of deep structures:
  - – Blood vessels
  - – Nerves
  - – Tendons
  - – Viscera
  - – Bone

6

Further treatment
Pain relief, antibiotics, tetanus shot

❶ Type of injury

Cuts and lacerations Cuts are caused by sharp objects. They are usually clean-edged and heal well. Lacerations are caused by blunt objects. They are more ragged, harder to repair, and are more prone to infection.

Abrasion Small abrasions (grazes) are common and require simple cleaning. Severe abrasions may result in considerable tissue loss and require surgery when ashore. These should be cleaned thoroughly to avoid "tattooing" (discoloured scarring) and antibiotics used if significant tissue loss has occurred.

Bruising A bruise (haematoma) may appear innocuous, but a collection of blood in the tissues may become infected, causing an abscess, which will require draining. Watch for signs of infection.

Bites These may be human or animal. They require very thorough cleaning and should always be treated with broad-spectrum antibiotics as they are very prone to infection.

Penetrating wounds Wounds of this type are difficult to assess on a boat, but injuries to organs, bone, tendons, nerves, or blood vessels beneath the wound are likely. Observe the casualty closely, and seek medical advice at the first opportunity.

Amputations Traumatic amputations of fingers and toes are not uncommon on boats. The casualty should be evacuated as soon as possible and the digit kept cool (not frozen). Again, seek medical advice as soon as possible. Traumatic amputation of a limb is life-threatening and a medical emergency.

❷ Assess severity

History The mechanism of injury may give an idea about extent and severity.

Important points in the history	
□ How did the accident happen? (knife, glass, energy involved)	□ Is there risk of contamination? (seawater is not necessarily sterile)
□ When and where did it happen?	□ Who else was involved?
□ Was the casualty crushed at all?	□ Date of last tetanus vaccination?

Examination Carry out the examination in a well-lit, secure place where you can take your time. Be thorough. Proper examination of a penetrating wound at sea is impossible, but attempt to examine to the bottom of any wound for contamination. Use local anaesthetic (see pp.184–85).

Important points in the examination	
□ Size and shape of wound	□ Signs of infection:
□ Contamination and foreign bodies	– Redness around the wound
□ Presence of pulses beyond injury	– Painful swelling
□ Signs of nerve damage:	– Swollen lymph nodes in groin, armpit
– Sensation	– Lymphangitis: Red streaks or lines
– Movement	spreading up the arm

❸ Control bleeding

□ Bleeding from a vein can be controlled by raising the limb above the heart.
□ Bleeding from an artery may spurt with the pulse and needs direct pressure to the wound or pressure on each side if direct pressure is too painful.
□ Only use pressure points (the pulses that are usually felt in the groin or armpit), tourniquets, or artery forceps if direct pressure does not work; perfusion to the distal part of the limb may be dangerously reduced, but this may be necessary.
□ Haemostatic dressings or powder can be used to control/stop major bleeding. Always use with direct pressure, not alone, or it won't work.
□ Tranexamic acid is effective in limiting major haemorrhage. Ideally, 4g IV injection or otherwise oral tablets. Use only with direct medical advice.

❹ Wound closure (see p.68)

□ Ideally, wounds should be closed within 12-24 hours.
□ Wound closure is an effective way of reducing blood loss.
□ Absorbable sutures are usually used to close layers of tissue below the skin. Use nonabsorbable sutures for the skin.
□ Sterile adhesive skin tape is effective and quick for small wounds, if the skin is dry.
□ Skin staples from a dedicated skin stapler are rapid and good for wet skin, but require a proper staple extractor.
□ Tissue adhesive (skin glue) is fast but useless if the skin is damp or under tension.
□ Healing will be improved, especially of large wounds, if the limb is immobilized to prevent stretching of the skin repair. The casualty should rest as much as possible.

❺ Complications

□ Infection is likely, and wounds should be inspected every 24-36 hours and re-dressed with a sterile dressing. Infection should be treated with broad-spectrum antibiotics as soon as it is suspected.
□ Infection may lead to reccurrence of bleeding a few days after the accident. Thorough cleaning of infected tissue is necessary (under local anaesthetic, which may be only partially effective). Seek medical advice if this occurs.
□ Foreign bodies (dirt, grit, etc.) may lead to infection if not removed immediately and may also cause discoloured scarring (tattooing) once the wound has healed.
□ Damage to structures below the skin may cause a wide variety of complications. If there is ongoing pain, loss of movement or sensation, or bleeding, seek medical advice regarding further treatment, particularly for penetrating wounds.

❻ Further treatment

□ Antibiotics are indicated for:
  - Heavily contaminated wounds
  - Any form of bite
  - Fractures where the bone comes through the skin
  - Traumatic amputation
  - Wounds that become infected

□ Pain relief is essential and should be given as soon as possible.
□ Local anaesthetic injection (infiltration) around wounds will help examination and repair (see pp.184-85).
□ Check that the person's tetanus vaccination is up to date.

HEAD INJURIES

Minor head injuries are common on boats, and recovery is usually quick and complete. Serious head injuries are more rare and usually grave, requiring urgent evacuation. The most important piece of advice about head injuries is to avoid them.

Following head injury, prompt and appropriate treatment may reduce severity and prevent deterioration of the brain due to lack of blood pressure or oxygen.

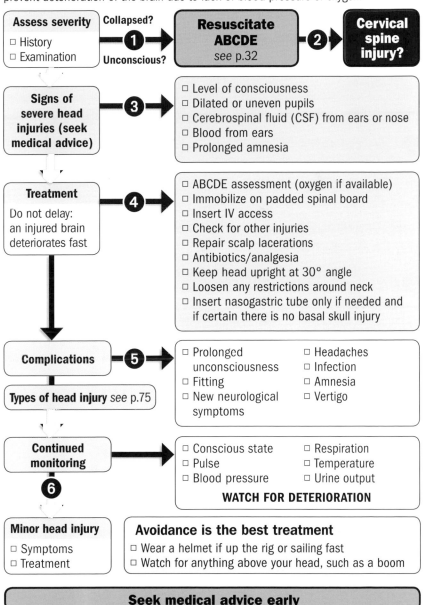

Assess severity
- □ History
- □ Examination

Collapsed? ➊
Unconscious?

Resuscitate ABCDE *see p.32* ➋

Cervical spine injury?

Signs of severe head injuries (seek medical advice) ➌
- □ Level of consciousness
- □ Dilated or uneven pupils
- □ Cerebrospinal fluid (CSF) from ears or nose
- □ Blood from ears
- □ Prolonged amnesia

Treatment
Do not delay: an injured brain deteriorates fast ➍
- □ ABCDE assessment (oxygen if available)
- □ Immobilize on padded spinal board
- □ Insert IV access
- □ Check for other injuries
- □ Repair scalp lacerations
- □ Antibiotics/analgesia
- □ Keep head upright at 30° angle
- □ Loosen any restrictions around neck
- □ Insert nasogastric tube only if needed and if certain there is no basal skull injury

Complications ➎

Types of head injury see p.75
- □ Prolonged unconsciousness
- □ Fitting
- □ New neurological symptoms
- □ Headaches
- □ Infection
- □ Amnesia
- □ Vertigo

Continued monitoring ➏
- □ Conscious state
- □ Pulse
- □ Blood pressure
- □ Respiration
- □ Temperature
- □ Urine output

WATCH FOR DETERIORATION

Minor head injury
- □ Symptoms
- □ Treatment

Avoidance is the best treatment
- □ Wear a helmet if up the rig or sailing fast
- □ Watch for anything above your head, such as a boom

Seek medical advice early

❶ History and examination

- ☐ ABCDE assessment (*see* page 32) takes priority over everything else.
- ☐ Take particular care of the neck (*see* 2, below).
- ☐ A conscious crew is reassuring but may deteriorate later.
- ☐ Get as much information as possible from other crew members.

Important points in the history	Important points in the examination
☐ How did the accident happen? ☐ Was there loss of consciousness? For how long? ☐ Does the casualty have loss of memory (amnesia) and for how long? ☐ Has the casualty been sick, or does he or she feel sick? ☐ Does the casualty have a headache?	☐ Level of consciousness (*see* below) ☐ Size and reactivity of pupils (*see* below) ☐ Weakness or paralysis of face or limbs ☐ Heart rate, blood pressure, respiratory rate

❷ Cervical spine (neck) injury

Spinal injuries are common with head injury. The bones of the neck may be broken and be unstable, but the spinal cord may still be intact. If in doubt, immobilize the cervical spine immobilization (*see* pp.164–65).

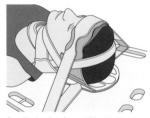

Cervical spine immobilization

❸ Signs of severe head injury

Level of consciousness In general, the worse the conscious level, the worse the head injury. A casualty may initially appear to be conscious after an injury but may deteriorate rapidly. Therefore, monitor conscious level frequently.

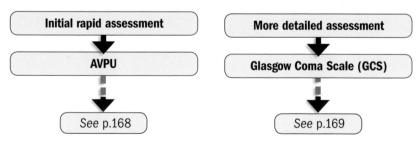

If the patient is less than "alert" on the AVPU scale, assess using GCS. Reassess every 15 minutes for at least the first few hours.
- ☐ GCS score 9–12: possible significant head injury
- ☐ GCS score <8: serious head injury
- ☐ Reduction in GCS score of 2 or more: serious deterioration

Seek medical advice early

Dilated or uneven pupils Pupils should normally be equal and reactive to light. A head injury may cause the pupils to be: unequal in size; unreactive to light; and dilated and unreactive.

Pupil size	Pupil response to light	Likely cause
 Both pupils equally dilated	Responsive equally	Fear, alcohol, drugs such as cocaine
 Both pupils equally constricted	Responsive equally	Bright light, drugs such as opiates or benzodiazepines
 Pupils uneven	Larger pupil unresponsive	Head injury, eye injury or direct drug contamination, such as with hyoscine hydrobromide (in anti-seasickness patches)
 Both pupils dilated	Both pupils unresponsive	Severe injury to head, death

Cerebrospinal fluid (CSF) or blood from the ears CSF is clear and looks similar to tears and nasal or mouth secretions. Bear this in mind when you see clear fluid around the head. Blood in the ears may have come from the inside, but it may also have run into the ears from scalp or facial wounds. If in any doubt, assume any clear fluid is CSF, and assume fluid in the ears has come from inside until proven otherwise.

Prolonged post-traumatic amnesia (PTA) A short period of loss of memory after an injury to the head is quite common. A period of amnesia greater than 30 minutes indicates a significant head injury.

④ Treatment

A casualty with a suspected head injury should be evacuated as soon as possible. Treatment on a boat remote from land is aimed at preventing complications. Once the casualty has been assessed for ABCDE, given oxygen if available, and immobilized on a padded, rigid board to protect potential spinal fractures and prevent pressure sores, it is important to look for other injuries (the secondary survey – see pp.34–35). **A patient who has received a head injury and who is also in shock is very likely to have another injury.**

☐ Scalp lacerations bleed heavily, and a lot of blood may be lost in a short time. Repair them as quickly as possible, by suturing, stapling, or gluing.

☐ IV fluids may be required to restore blood pressure to normal.

☐ The patient should be kept head–up if possible, which can be achieved by tilting the rigid board. If there are any tight restrictions around the neck, such as a dry-suit seal, these should be removed. These manoeuvres help to reduce pressure in the brain.

☐ DO NOT put in a nasogastric tube if there are signs of a basal skull fracture (black eyes, blood, or CSF from ears or nose). In these cases there is a danger that the tube may end up in the brain. Ask for medical advice before attempting.

☐ Avoid giving morphine to head injured patients. Regular paracetamol and codeine may be used and should not reduce the conscious level.

☐ If there is suspicion of a skull fracture, give antibiotics.

☐ Tranexamic acid can be used to limit bleeding within the skull, but must only be used under direct medical advice.

⑤ Complications

Medical advice should have been sought by this stage and MUST be sought if there are any signs of complications. Any sign of deterioration in the casualty's conscious level or new signs of paralysis of the face or one side of the body are ominous and the casualty must be evacuated urgently. Managing an unconscious casualty on a boat for a prolonged period is a complex and difficult task. The process is described on pp.36–38.

Fitting Seizures are common after relatively minor head injuries, and should stop by themselves after a minute or so. Recurrent, prolonged fitting, with fits lasting longer than 1–2 minutes, is much more concerning and should be treated (see p.40).

Signs of infection Temperature, flushing, or signs of meningism (see p.117), such as photophobia (intolerance of bright light), stiffness in the neck, and headache, are very serious because they may indicate an infection. Administer IV broad-spectrum antibiotics.

Vertigo The whirling sensations associated with vertigo are common following a head injury, and these symptoms may be treated using either prochlorperazine or cyclizine.

Headaches Use nonsedating painkillers if possible. Worsening of a headache may indicate worsening of the head injury, so seek medical advice.

6 Minor head injuries

Symptoms
- Dizziness
- Headache
- Difficulty concentrating
- Vomiting (no more than 3 times)
- Tiredness

Treatment
Nonsedating painkillers for headache.
Prochlorperazine or cyclizine for dizziness if bad.

Rest for a few days as necessary, avoiding strenuous activities.
Watch for deterioration in conscious level or vital signs.

Outlook
Symptoms should last only a few days at most. Seek medical advice if they persist longer than this.

Types of head injuries

Closed Closed head injuries are the most common type. The skull of the casualty is not fractured (or there is only a minor fracture) and the brain is not exposed. These injuries are usually caused by a blunt blow to the head, such as a collision with the boom or the spinnaker pole, or falling down stairs.

Open Less common than closed injuries, open injuries are usually more serious. The brain is exposed, which may be obvious to the untrained eye, but will sometimes be difficult to assess in cases of basal skull fracture. Open head injuries are usually caused by sharp objects or small, blunt objects, such as stanchions, and carry a high risk of infection. There are three types of open head injury:

- Penetrating: when a sharp object, such as a marlinspike, goes through the skull and into the brain.
- Compound depressed skull fracture: caused by collision with a small, solid object such as a stanchion top. A piece of the skull is pushed into the brain.
- Basal skull fracture: a type of fracture running across the base of the skull and opening up a communication between the inside of the casualty's skull and the tubes of the ears or nose.

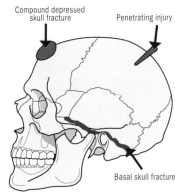

Open head injuries

Primary injury This term refers to the direct result of the blow to the head. For example, the primary injury could be a skull fracture, damage to the brain tissue itself, or bleeding in the brain.

Secondary injury Following a primary injury, the brain may deteriorate due to lack of blood flow or oxygen; this is secondary injury. Although resources on a boat may be limited, a few straightforward actions, such as establishing an airway and immobilizing the neck, may reduce the severity of secondary injury.

NECK AND SPINAL INJURIES

Fortunately, spinal injuries are rare on boats – back strains and sprains are much more common. However, very occasionally, what looks like a minor injury is in fact very serious, so if there is any doubt, immobilize the casualty and seek medical advice. Damage to the spinal cord is dire and usually irreversible, so make every effort to protect an injured or unstable spine: do not move the patient without spinal immobilization.

Severity of injury is likely to be greater in accidents involving more energy, such as falling from a height. Alcohol and obvious injuries such as broken limbs and open wounds might divert attention from a spinal injury.

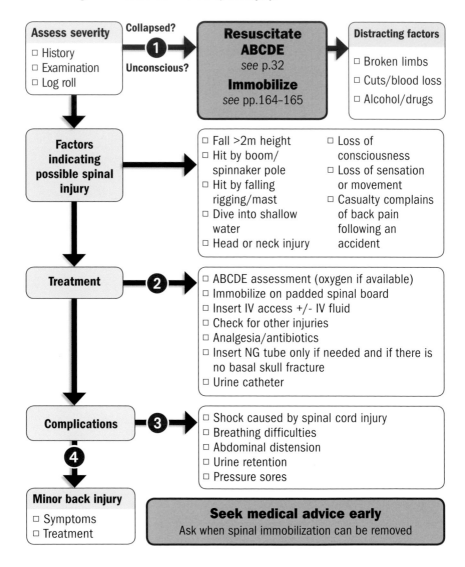

Assess severity
- ☐ History
- ☐ Examination
- ☐ Log roll

Collapsed?

1

Unconscious?

Resuscitate ABCDE
see p.32
Immobilize
see pp.164–165

Distracting factors
- ☐ Broken limbs
- ☐ Cuts/blood loss
- ☐ Alcohol/drugs

Factors indicating possible spinal injury
- ☐ Fall >2m height
- ☐ Hit by boom/ spinnaker pole
- ☐ Hit by falling rigging/mast
- ☐ Dive into shallow water
- ☐ Head or neck injury
- ☐ Loss of consciousness
- ☐ Loss of sensation or movement
- ☐ Casualty complains of back pain following an accident

Treatment

2
- ☐ ABCDE assessment (oxygen if available)
- ☐ Immobilize on padded spinal board
- ☐ Insert IV access +/- IV fluid
- ☐ Check for other injuries
- ☐ Analgesia/antibiotics
- ☐ Insert NG tube only if needed and if there is no basal skull fracture
- ☐ Urine catheter

Complications

3
- ☐ Shock caused by spinal cord injury
- ☐ Breathing difficulties
- ☐ Abdominal distension
- ☐ Urine retention
- ☐ Pressure sores

4

Minor back injury
- ☐ Symptoms
- ☐ Treatment

Seek medical advice early
Ask when spinal immobilization can be removed

❶ History and examination

□ ABCDE assessment (*see* p.32) takes priority over everything else.
□ Anyone with a head injury may well have a spinal injury as well.
□ A proper examination for possible neck and spinal injuries will require a log roll (*see* p.163), four people will be needed to turn the casualty and one to examine the back.

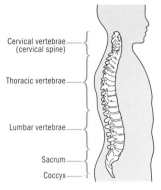

Parts of the spine

Important points in the history

□ How did the accident happen?
□ Where is the pain?
□ Are there any symptoms of nerve damage? – Numbness
              – Pins and needles
              – Loss of movement
□ Any previous history of back pain or injuries?

Important points in the examination
Look Obvious injuries to head, neck, spine; swelling, bruising **Feel** Tenderness, steps in spine, can the casualty feel touch and pain? **Move** Can patient move body and limbs? If neck injured, do not move it **Document** Tone, power, sensation for all limbs and the main body

❷ Treatment

A casualty with a suspected spinal injury must be evacuated as soon as possible.
Immobilization (*see* pp.164–165) The whole body must be immobilized as effectively as possible using a semi-rigid collar and a padded board.
IV access and fluid Casualty may have low blood pressure and need IV fluid.
Nasogastric (NG) tube, urinary catheter (see pp.186–88) An immobilized patient may be kept hydrated by an NG tube and will need a urinary catheter.
Analgesia, antibiotics Pain relief to settle the casualty; antibiotics for an open wound.

❸ Complications

□ Low blood pressure (shock) may be caused by relaxation of blood vessels due to spinal cord damage. Seek medical advice about how much fluid to give.
□ If the spinal cord injury is high in the chest or in the neck, the casualty may not be able to breathe properly. This is an ominous problem on a boat. Give oxygen if available and follow ABC assessment if the patient stops breathing (*see* p.30).
□ The gut may stop working, and the casualty may vomit. Once an NG tube is in place, aspirate all the stomach contents out initially to reduce the risk.

❹ Minor back injuries

Symptoms A minor back injury will cause localized pain that is worse on straining or coughing. Pain may extend down the leg (sciatica) and posture may be abnormal.
Treatments Administer pain relief to allow mobilization and prevent stiffness. If the casualty has sciatica, advise rest and seek medical advice. Care should be taken with the posture during vigorous activities such as winching and helming.

FACIAL INJURIES

Flogging sails and sheets, the boom, the spinnaker pole, and trips ashore when in port can all result in facial injuries. These may look bad, but they often turn out to be minor.

Bony injuries, however, may be difficult to detect. The immediate risk with facial fractures is damage to the airway, which can result in death within minutes; various manoeuvres will minimize this risk. A less obvious danger is swelling, which may compromise the airway hours after the initial injury. Head and neck injuries often occur at the same time, so the ABCDE approach to assessing the casualty is essential.

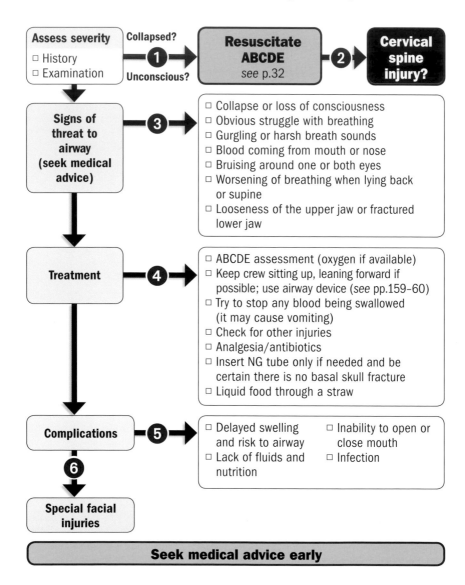

Assess severity
- □ History
- □ Examination

Collapsed?

Unconscious?

① →

Resuscitate ABCDE
see p.32

② →

Cervical spine injury?

Signs of threat to airway (seek medical advice)

③ →

- □ Collapse or loss of consciousness
- □ Obvious struggle with breathing
- □ Gurgling or harsh breath sounds
- □ Blood coming from mouth or nose
- □ Bruising around one or both eyes
- □ Worsening of breathing when lying back or supine
- □ Looseness of the upper jaw or fractured lower jaw

Treatment

④ →

- □ ABCDE assessment (oxygen if available)
- □ Keep crew sitting up, leaning forward if possible; use airway device (see pp.159–60)
- □ Try to stop any blood being swallowed (it may cause vomiting)
- □ Check for other injuries
- □ Analgesia/antibiotics
- □ Insert NG tube only if needed and be certain there is no basal skull fracture
- □ Liquid food through a straw

Complications

⑤ →

- □ Delayed swelling and risk to airway
- □ Lack of fluids and nutrition
- □ Inability to open or close mouth
- □ Infection

⑥

Special facial injuries

Seek medical advice early

❶ History and examination

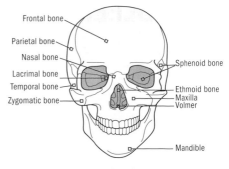

- ☐ Be aware that anyone with a facial injury may well have sustained additional injuries, particularly to the head and neck.
- ☐ It might be difficult to find out exactly what happened from the crew member who has a facial injury, so collect as much information as you can from witnesses.

Frontal bone
Parietal bone
Nasal bone
Lacrimal bone
Temporal bone
Zygomatic bone
Sphenoid bone
Ethmoid bone
Maxilla
Volmer
Mandible

Bones of the face

Important points in the history

- ☐ How did the accident happen?
- ☐ Was there any loss of consciousness? For how long?
- ☐ Any difficulty breathing?
- ☐ Any problems with vision (double vision, for example)?

Important points in the examination

Look Obvious injuries to face, deformed nose, swellings, blood
Feel Tenderness over cheeks, jaw, steps in bone edges, crepitus
Move Ask casualty to open and close mouth. Do the teeth line up? Is the upper jaw loose?

---

❷ Cervical spine (neck) injury

Spinal injuries commonly accompany head injuries. Keep in mind that the bones of the neck may be broken and unstable, but the spinal cord may still be intact. If you are in any doubt at all about the nature of the injury, immobilize the cervical spine (see pp.164–65).

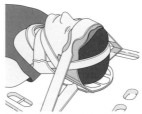

Cervical spine immobilization

---

❸ Signs of threat to airway

Any fracture to the middle of the face or jaw (mandible) is a possible risk to the airway, because the fractured piece of face or jaw may fall back into the airway and partially or entirely block it.

The casualty may be struggling and making harsh or gurgling sounds when breathing in. Other signs such as pain, swelling, bilateral black eyes, and blood from the mouth may also be caused by facial fractures.

If the casualty is conscious, they will be able to describe their difficulties with breathing and whether sitting up and leaning forward eases them. Being upright and leaning forward helps to clear the airway by allowing the broken part of the face or jaw to "hang forward", clearing the airway.

A fracture through the mid-part of the face, above the upper jaw (through the maxilla), may result in the upper jaw being "loose". Test this by holding the upper front teeth firmly with the fingers and gently trying to move the upper jaw in and out. Only do this once, as repetitions will cause pain, bleeding, and further swelling.

❹ Immediate treatment

- ☐ A casualty with a suspected facial fracture should be evacuated as soon as possible.
- ☐ If the casualty is conscious but having difficulty breathing, try to keep them sitting up and leaning forward.
- ☐ Lie unconscious casualties in the recovery position if you are sure there are no spine injuries (see pp.162–63).
- ☐ An airway adjunct, such as a oropharyngeal airway, may be needed (see p.159), but insert very gently. Do not insert a nasopharyngeal airway unless absolutely certain there is no basal-skull or mid-face fracture.
- ☐ Either drain blood from the mouth in the recovery position or use a suction device if available. Blood in the stomach is a strong stimulus for vomiting. Any vomit may end up in the lungs.
- ☐ Use nonsedating painkillers – paracetamol, nonsteroidal anti-inflammatory drugs (NSAIDs): NSAIDs may reduce swelling.
- ☐ Insert a nasogastric (NG) tube only if really needed, and then only if you are absolutely sure there is no basal-skull or mid-face fracture. Seek medical advice.
- ☐ Swallowing or chewing may be painful and difficult. It may be impossible to close the mouth. Liquid food through an NG tube or straw may be required.
- ☐ Use antibiotics for lacerations, continual blood in the mouth, or a temperature.

❺ Complications

- ☐ Swelling after a fracture may worsen for a few days after the injury. Get medical advice if there is any doubt regarding the airway and make plans to evacuate.
- ☐ If oral fluid intake is not sufficient, rehydrate by another route (see pp.170–71).
- ☐ Fractures or dislocations of the jaw or cheek bones may prevent the mouth from opening or closing. A mouth which is jammed open is painful and potentially dangerous. Get medical advice and evacuate as soon as possible.
- ☐ Infection is a significant risk with facial fractures, because fractures that run into the mouth, airway, or sinuses are impossible to diagnose on a boat. Any suspected fracture should be treated with antibiotics until evacuation.

❻ Specific facial injuries

Lacerations of the face and lips
Facial lacerations bleed heavily and look horrible before they are cleaned up. For cosmetic reasons, take care when suturing, using sterile tape, or gluing. If the lips have been lacerated, realign the lip edges as accurately as possible during suturing. Clean the wound thoroughly using local anaesthetic (see pp.184–85). Use interrupted sutures with the finest thread possible and antibiotics for large or dirty wounds (see p.178).

Tongue injuries
The teeth may lacerate the tongue in a blow to the face. If there is blood in the mouth, examine the tongue carefully. Get medical advice if there is a significant injury to the tongue and keep the casualty sitting up to reduce any swelling that may compromise the airway.

Fractured nose

Nose breaks cause copious bleeding, which may be stopped by squeezing the soft part of the nose firmly. After getting medical advice, it might be necessary to pack the nose with a gauze strip soaked in adrenaline or petroleum jelly. A bent nose may be firmly realigned immediately (if the casualty allows), before swelling occurs. A haematoma in the septum should be drained carefully under local anaesthesia, otherwise the haematoma may in turn cause tissue death.

Fractures of the cheek bone (maxilla)

Symptoms and signs:

□ A black eye
□ Double vision
□ Possible pain in the eye
□ Difficulty opening mouth/chewing
□ "Step" on lower ridge of eye socket

Analgesia and a soft diet will reduce discomfort. Arrange to evacuate the casualty as soon as possible.

Fractures of the mid-face

A large amount of force is required to cause such a fracture, so other injuries are likely. Seek medical advice urgently and arrange for evacuation as soon as possible. Symptoms and signs:

□ Difficulty with the airway and breathing
□ Bilateral black eyes
□ A loose upper jaw
□ A step in the teeth of the upper jaw
□ Difficulty in opening the mouth

Assess and support the airway. This may be very difficult in an unconscious patient and may prove impossible on a boat, without specialist equipment and immediate skilled help. Do your best. Other supportive treatments are outlined on pp.36–38.

Dislocated mandible

Dislocation can be caused by a blow to the jaw or by opening the mouth very wide – during a yawn, for example. It then becomes impossible to close the mouth. The jaw may be twisted off to one side, in which case only one of the joints is dislocated. The dislocation should be reduced as soon as possible. Seek medical advice. You may need to sedate the casualty before he or she relaxes enough for you to get the jaw back in to place.

Fractured mandible

A reasonable amount of force is required to fracture the mandible, and severe fractures may be life-threatening. Seek medical advice urgently and evacuate. Symptoms and signs:

□ Difficulty with airway and breathing
□ Obvious deformity of jaw line
□ "Step" in the teeth of the lower jaw
□ Difficulty opening the mouth
□ Swelling along jaw and up side of head

Barton bandage
A Barton bandage passes around the head three times, as shown above, and is secured at the top.

Assess and support the airway, which may prove as difficult as with a mid-face fracture. The mandible can be immobilized by wiring the teeth of the lower jaw to the teeth of the upper jaw, but this requires skill and an extremely brave patient. A Barton bandage (see illustration above), which is less invasive and easier than wiring, can also be used. Be prepared to cut it off quickly if the patient vomits.

EYE INJURIES

The eyeball is relatively well protected in its bony socket, with only about 20 per cent of the eyeball surface visible. Direct eye injuries are thus rare, but potentially sight-threatening. Injuries to the mid-face and cheek bone may be associated with eye injuries. Examine any lacerations closely.

Crew members who normally wear glasses should ideally use plastic lenses to avoid lacerations caused by shattered glass fragments. Contact lenses can cause problems in a marine environment, particularly in freezing wind and salt spray conditions.

History

- If eye is injured, how and when?
- Duration of symptoms?
- Any history of foreign bodies in the eye?
- Painful or painless eye?
- Previous eye/vision problems
- Eye surgery in the past (cataract/laser)?
- Contact lenses or glasses?
- Diabetes or glaucoma?

Examination

This needs to be done in a safe and stable place, such as in a bunk. The area should be well lit, with a head torch if necessary, and the casualty provided with painkillers.

Look

- Obvious bruising, swelling, lacerations
- Foreign bodies under lids or inside the eye
- Pupil size and reaction to light
- Reddened sclera
- Tears streaming from the eye
- Blood inside the eye. You may see blood in front of the iris
- Examine the cornea using magnifying glass and fluorescein eye drops – these glow in bright blue light, showing up abrasions. Put local anaesthetic (tetracaine) drops in the eye first
- Look inside eyelids: gently pull lower lid down; turn back upper lid (*see* opposite).
- Compare one side with the other

Feel

- Bony steps around the edge of the eye socket (orbit)
- Firmness of the eyeball (gently) to get an idea of intraocular pressure

Move

- Ask the casualty to look at your finger held about 30cm away
- Move the finger up and down and from side to side slowly, keeping the head still
- Ask about double vision, and watch eye movements closely
- Document any pain

Visual Acuity

- Ask the casualty whether their visual acuity is normal
- Test vision by reading small text from a book at normal distance

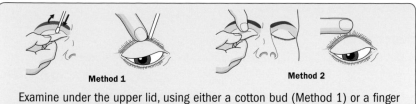

Method 1 **Method 2**

Examine under the upper lid, using either a cotton bud (Method 1) or a finger (Method 2) to roll back the lid.

Immediate treatment

Seek medical advice for any injury in which the eyesight is affected, for penetrating injuries, and for chemical burns, or if you are worried. Assess for other facial injuries (*see* p.78).

Pain relief

Orally	Other injuries may have occurred and the casualty will need to be comfortable to allow examination
To the eye	Tetracaine (0.5% or 1%) local anaesthetic eye drops, a few drops inside each lower lid. The local anaesthetic action will last up to an hour or so. Pad the eye if still painful after examination

Antibiotics If in doubt, apply antibiotic drops or ointment: drops are easier to use; ointment lasts longer and lubricates the eye nicely, but blurs the vision. Chloramphenicol is the usual broad-spectrum antibiotic used for the eyes. For penetrating injuries, and where there is blood or foreign bodies in the eye, use oral antibiotics as well.

Eye pads Padding a painful eye will reduce pain. Do not apply undue pressure and do not pad both eyes at the same time unless you have to. Make sure the eyelids are shut, particularly if the eye is anaesthetized. Padding may scratch a partly open eye.

Foreign bodies Remove any visible foreign bodies immediately by flushing out with sterile normal saline or water or by gently using a cotton bud.

Chemicals Flush with copius sterile water or normal saline as soon as possible after the accident, using a plastic bag with a small hole in it. Continue for at least 10 minutes or, if the chemical was an alkali, for at least 30 minutes.

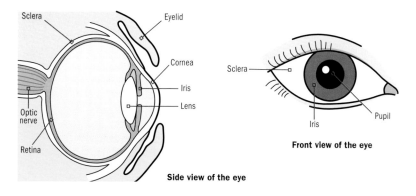

Side view of the eye

Front view of the eye

Specific eye problems

Eyelid laceration
□ This is a serious injury, often accompanied by other injures to the eye itself.
□ If the eye is left exposed, corneal damage and infection are more likely to occur.
□ Seek medical advice regarding repair.

Symptoms and signs	Treatment
□ Examine eye after local anaesthetic drops □ Look carefully for other injuries, particularly if high energy involved □ Look for foreign bodies in the eye and eyelid □ Take particular care if the eyelid margin is lacerated	□ Apply firm but gentle pressure to stop bleeding □ Remove foreign bodies □ Antibiotic ointment or drops and oral broad-spectrum antibiotics to stop orbital cellulitis □ Get medical advice if you plan to attempt a repair yourself □ Pad the eye and use artificial tears if the cornea is left exposed

Corneal abrasion
Corneal abrasion is caused by a foreign body on the surface of the eye, an object hitting the open eye, or lack of care with an anaesthetized eye.

Symptoms and signs	Treatment
□ Painful eye □ Feels like a foreign body in the eye □ Abrasion may be seen in a magnifying glass, with the help of fluorescein staining and a blue light	□ Flush the eye to remove any foreign bodies that remain □ Use local anaesthetic drops for pain □ Administer oral pain relief if there is an accompanying headache □ Use antibiotic ointment or drops to lubricate and soothe the abrasion □ Pad the eye if particularly painful

Foreign body
The object may be under the eyelids or may even have penetrated the eyeball itself (see penetrating eye injury, below).

Symptoms and signs	Treatment
□ Mechanism of injury? □ Examine eye after local anaesthetic and fluorescein drops (see p.117) □ Examine under the upper and lower eyelids (see pp.82–83) □ The eye will produce a lot of tears	□ Pain relief with local anaesthetic eyedrops □ If obvious, remove foreign body with (clean) finger or cotton bud □ Flush eye with sterile water or normal saline. Use a clean plastic bag with a small hole in it if no syringe is available. Boil water and fully cool if nothing else is available □ Antibiotic ointment or drops to soothe and lubricate the eye

Chemical burn

- Burns with alkali chemicals are generally worse than those with acids.
- Medical advice is required for all chemical burns as soon as possible.
- Identify which chemical was involved (for example, battery acid).

Symptoms and signs	Treatment
- Red, painful eye - Look for chemical burn to surrounding face - Eyesight might be blurred - One or both eyes may be involved	- Start flushing eye immediately before chemical penetrates eye - Use the cleanest water/normal saline available urgently (sterile preferably) - Flush for at least 30 minutes or longer - Antibiotic ointment for lubrication and comfort (also use artificial tears) - Local anaesthetic drops if very painful

Nonpenetrating eye injury

- A blunt blow to the face that may cause other facial injuries.
- Weakest point of orbit is the floor (below the eye), and this may "blow out" into the space (sinus) below.

Symptoms and signs	Treatment
- Mechanism of injury? - Black eye, swelling, bruising - Pain on eye movement - Injury to eye itself - An eyeball that looks sunken - Compare with the other side - Assess for other injuries	- Thoroughly examine eye before swelling prevents eye opening - Treat other injuries - Consider local anaesthetic drops/antibiotic drops to eye if painful - Pad/cover the eye if double vision causing distress - Consider ice pack for swelling/bruising

Penetrating eye injury

- This may be obvious, but might be difficult to see with small objects entering through the cornea – any hole closes quickly.
- The energy involved in the accident is important; high-speed metal fragments are more likely to penetrate the eyeball.
- Seek medical advice immediately, as eyesight may be threatened.

Symptoms and signs	Treatment
- Mechanism of injury? - Painful red eye - Irregular pupil - Decreased vision - Visible foreign body in/behind cornea - Laceration of cornea/sclera - Soft eye - Leakage of eye contents	- Do not remove object impaled in eye - Guard against impaled object being pushed further in - Antibiotic ointment or drops - Local anaesthetic drops - Oral broad-spectrum antibiotics - Pad over eye, with shield to prevent impaled object moving - Seek medical advice immediately

CHEST INJURIES

On a boat, chest injuries tend to be blunt traumas caused by falling onto objects. Note that about 50 per cent of injuries happen below deck: falls onto table edges, for example. Penetrating chest injuries are rare and usually more serious.

Severe bruising of the chest wall is indistinguishable from fractured ribs. Both are disabling and are treated in a similar manner. However, the major concern about chest injury is the possibility of lung or heart involvement. Pre-existing lung or heart disease aggravates the problem.

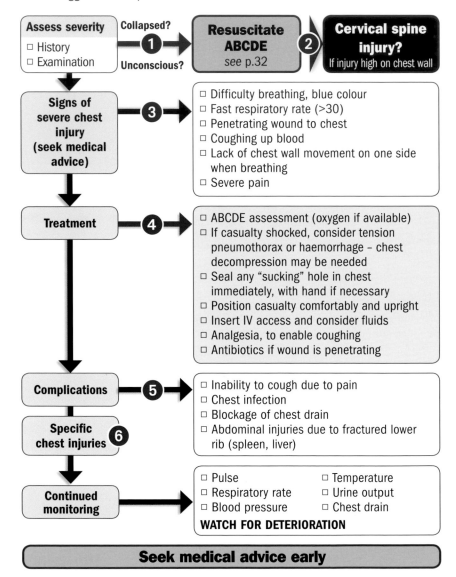

Assess severity
- □ History
- □ Examination

Collapsed?

1

Unconscious?

Resuscitate ABCDE
see p.32

2

Cervical spine injury?
If injury high on chest wall

Signs of severe chest injury (seek medical advice)

3

- □ Difficulty breathing, blue colour
- □ Fast respiratory rate (>30)
- □ Penetrating wound to chest
- □ Coughing up blood
- □ Lack of chest wall movement on one side when breathing
- □ Severe pain

Treatment

4

- □ ABCDE assessment (oxygen if available)
- □ If casualty shocked, consider tension pneumothorax or haemorrhage – chest decompression may be needed
- □ Seal any "sucking" hole in chest immediately, with hand if necessary
- □ Position casualty comfortably and upright
- □ Insert IV access and consider fluids
- □ Analgesia, to enable coughing
- □ Antibiotics if wound is penetrating

Complications

5

Specific chest injuries

6

- □ Inability to cough due to pain
- □ Chest infection
- □ Blockage of chest drain
- □ Abdominal injuries due to fractured lower rib (spleen, liver)

Continued monitoring

- □ Pulse
- □ Respiratory rate
- □ Blood pressure
- □ Temperature
- □ Urine output
- □ Chest drain

WATCH FOR DETERIORATION

Seek medical advice early

❶ History and examination

- ABCDE assessment (*see* p.32) takes first priority
- **Take special care of the neck if there is an injury high on the chest wall**
- Blue skin colouring around mouth is a very bad sign. Seek medical advice immediately
- Anticipate problems with breathing, pulse, and blood pressure
- Get as much information as possible from other crew about what happened

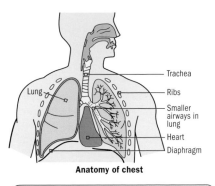

Anatomy of chest

Trachea
Ribs
Smaller airways in lung
Heart
Diaphragm
Lung

Important points in the history

- How did the accident happen (mechanism of injury)?
- Shortness of breath
- Pain in the chest
  - Location?
  - What makes it worse or better?
- Coughing up blood, sputum?
- Previous heart or lung disease (asthma/bronchitis)?
- Other injuries?

Important points in the examination

Look
- Appearance of casualty (blue/white)
- Obvious injuries to chest
- Look for difference in chest wall movement between each side

Feel
- Tenderness over chest wall
- Position of trachea (windpipe)

Listen
- Harsh or gurgling breath sounds
- Breath sounds in the chest (with a stethoscope)

Document Breathing rate/vital signs

❷ Cervical spine (neck) injury

Injuries high on the chest wall may be associated with injuries to the cervical spine. The bones of the neck may be broken and unstable, but the spinal cord may still be intact. If you are in any doubt at all, immobilize the cervical spine with a semi-rigid collar and a spinal board (*see* pp.164–165).

❸ Signs of severe chest injury

- The casualty may be struggling to breathe and have a high respiratory rate.
- Low blood pressure may be caused by loss of blood into the chest cavity (haemothorax) or by pressurized air in the chest cavity, compressing the lungs, heart, and blood vessels (*see* tension pneumothorax, pp.88–89).
- Any penetrating wound to the chest is serious and may have damaged lung, heart, and blood vessels and even abdominal organs.
- Coughing up blood indicates damage to both the lung and blood vessels.
- Lack of movement of one side of the chest in comparison with the other indicates one side does not function properly, probably due to blood or air in the chest cavity. The trachea, which should be in the centreline may be shifted to the opposite side.
- Pain is subjective: a stoic casualty may in fact have a serious injury.

④ Immediate treatment

If the casualty is having obvious difficulty with breathing, or has blue lips or fingers, seek medical advice immediately, and start to arrange for immediate evacuation if possible. Use oxygen if available.

Chest decompression Urgent decompresssion may be needed for suspected pneumothorax or haemothorax (see below and see p.180).

Sucking chest wound This type of wound should be sealed over urgently, even using a gloved hand, until a proper seal can be made (see pp.178–79).

Positioning The lungs generally work better in an upright position. This may be more comfortable, and the casualty should be wedged in place so they remain upright despite the rolling of the boat.

IV fluid May be required if the chest injury is serious or the blood pressure low. Seek medical advice regarding the amount of fluid.

Analgesia Coughing/deep breathing may not be possible because of the pain. Regular paracetamol, NSAIDs, and codeine may all be necessary. Morphine may be necessary to adequately control the pain – seek medical advice before using.

Antibiotics Use antibiotics for any penetrating, open chest wound, or if the casualty runs a temperature and starts to cough up green sputum.

⑤ Complications

Cough Inability to cough due to pain is serious. Secretions and any blood from the injury will pool in the lungs, leading to infection and making breathing more difficult. The casualty must be encouraged to breath deeply and cough for at least one good session every hour. Support damaged ribs with hands while doing this.

Chest infection Any sign of chest infection (temperature and/or yellow-green sputum) should be treated with antibiotics.

Blocked chest drain If a chest drain has been inserted, monitor the casualty very closely. Chest drains block easily, especially if there is blood in the chest. Pressure in the chest may rise again, possibly causing the casualty to collapse. Use a syringe to flush the drain with sterile normal saline or water.

Abdominal injury The lower ribs overlie the upper abdomen, and fractures of these ribs may damage the liver, spleen, and other organs.

⑥ Specific chest injuries

Pneumothorax

This condition occurs when there is air inside the chest but outside the lungs. It may occur spontaneously or may be caused by a blunt injury "bursting" the lung, a fractured rib piercing the lung, or a penetrating wound to the chest. If it is small, it has little or no effect on the circulation, and only makes breathing a little difficult. If it becomes very large, it may cause the lungs and heart to "collapse" (a "tension pneumothorax"). The chest must be decompressed quickly.

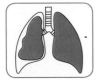

Small pneumothorax
Air collects between lung and chest wall

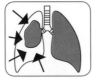

Tension pneumothorax
Air collects and pushes on lung and heart

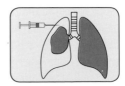

Immediate treatment
Insert needle and decompress

Symptoms and signs	Treatment
☐ Difficulty in breathing ☐ Low blood pressure ☐ The side of the chest not moving (may be difficult to identify) contains the air ☐ The trachea may be shifted away from the side of the chest with air in it ☐ Reduced breath sounds on the side of the chest with air in it	☐ Without delay, insert a needle or cannula between the ribs in the upper chest on the affected side (see p.180). ☐ A hiss of air may be heard when the needle enters the chest ☐ Insert a chest drain afterward if available (see pp.181–182)

Haemothorax

Damage to the ribs or blood vessels in the chest may cause bleeding, and the blood may accumulate inside the chest. A significant amount of blood (over 2L) may accumulate, causing the casualty to be shocked and the lung to be compressed.

Symptoms and signs	Treatment
☐ Difficulty in breathing ☐ Casualty may be shocked (low blood pressure) ☐ Faint breath sounds on affected side	☐ If you suspect a haemothorax, seek medical advice ☐ Insert IV line and give fluid ☐ Insert chest drain if available

Sucking chest wound

A sucking chest wound may cause deterioration in lung function and there may also be bleeding in to the chest that is not obvious externally.

Symptoms and signs	Treatment
☐ Casualty may be distressed, struggling with breathing, have blue lips, low blood pressure ☐ Obvious hissing/gurgling of air through a chest wound when breathing ☐ Harsh breath sounds on affected side	☐ Cover the hole immediately with a dressing (leaving one side unsealed) or with a gloved hand ☐ Insert chest drain though hole if possible (see pp.181–182) ☐ Seek medical advice

Broken ribs and chest wall bruising

Severe bruising and fractured ribs are indistinguishable on a boat, but both require rest and adequate pain relief. Broken ribs take up to 6 weeks to heal.

Symptoms and signs	Treatment
☐ Tenderness over chest wall at site ☐ Pain at fracture site if centre of chest is pushed in (be gentle) ☐ The broken ends of bone may be felt grating against each other (crepitus) ☐ A section of chest wall may move in instead of out when the casualty takes a breath in (a "flail" segment)	☐ Analgesia to enable the casualty to breath deeply and cough ☐ If a flail chest is suspected, give oxygen if possible and seek medical advice ☐ Do not bind the chest ☐ Keep comfortable in a bunk, but mobilize as soon as conditions allow

ABDOMINAL INJURIES

Injury to the organs in the abdomen may not cause symptoms at first and may be overlooked if there are other injuries. The main abdominal injuries are perforation of the bowel, bruising of the internal organs, and internal haemorrhage (often from tears to the liver and spleen). These injuries may result in infection and shock, causing the bowels to stop working. The kidneys are quite well protected, but they may be damaged by penetrating injury or severe blow to the flank.

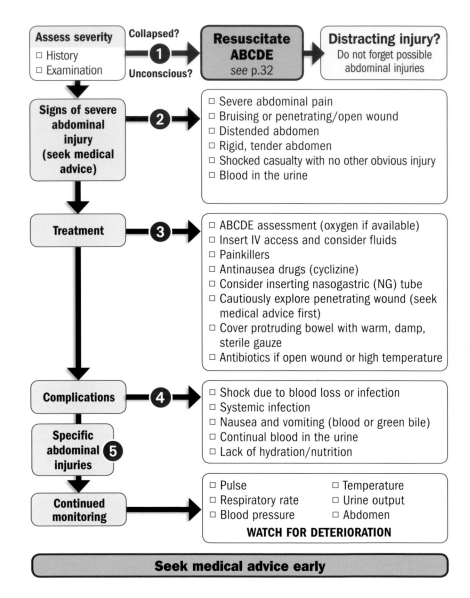

Assess severity
- History
- Examination

Collapsed?

Unconscious?

1

Resuscitate ABCDE
see p.32

Distracting injury?
Do not forget possible abdominal injuries

Signs of severe abdominal injury (seek medical advice)

2
- Severe abdominal pain
- Bruising or penetrating/open wound
- Distended abdomen
- Rigid, tender abdomen
- Shocked casualty with no other obvious injury
- Blood in the urine

Treatment

3
- ABCDE assessment (oxygen if available)
- Insert IV access and consider fluids
- Painkillers
- Antinausea drugs (cyclizine)
- Consider inserting nasogastric (NG) tube
- Cautiously explore penetrating wound (seek medical advice first)
- Cover protruding bowel with warm, damp, sterile gauze
- Antibiotics if open wound or high temperature

Complications

4
- Shock due to blood loss or infection
- Systemic infection
- Nausea and vomiting (blood or green bile)
- Continual blood in the urine
- Lack of hydration/nutrition

Specific abdominal injuries **5**

Continued monitoring
- Pulse
- Respiratory rate
- Blood pressure
- Temperature
- Urine output
- Abdomen

WATCH FOR DETERIORATION

Seek medical advice early

❶ History and examination

☐ Internal injuries may not be obvious at first, so reassess often if casualty is unwell.
☐ Remember to look at the back of the casualty.
☐ Penetrating injuries in the chest below the nipples may penetrate the abdomen.
☐ Lower rib fractures may damage the spleen or liver.

Important points in the history

☐ How did the accident happen (mechanism of injury)?
☐ Site and severity of pain?
☐ Any nausea, vomiting?
☐ Any blood or bile in vomit?
☐ Any blood in stool (may be red or tarry black) or urine (may be red or faintly pink)?

Important points in the examination

Look
☐ Abdominal wounds or bruising (look around the back)
☐ Abdominal distension
☐ Old operation scars (appendix, hernia)
Feel
☐ Any masses in the abdomen
☐ Tenderness, rigidity
Listen
☐ Bowel sounds (over lower right side)
Document On abdominal chart

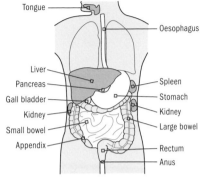

Abdominal organs

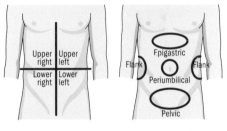

Abdominal quadrants   **Abdominal regions**

❷ Signs of severe abdominal injury

☐ The casualty may be sweaty and cold, from both the effects of pain and blood loss.
☐ A rigid, tense abdomen is a sign of serious injury.
☐ Any penetrating wound is serious and may have damaged many internal organs.
☐ The site and severity of pain gives an indication of which internal organs are damaged (*see* diagram above) and the possible severity of injury. Remember that people have different pain thresholds and also that the site of pain may be misleading. If in any doubt, monitor the casualty closely for signs of deterioration.
☐ Bruising of the abdomen may be difficult to see initially. If in doubt, re-examine the casualty every hour or so. Remember to examine the back for penetrating wounds and bruising. Flank bruising may indicate kidney injury.
☐ The abdomen may look normal at first, then become distended over a few hours.
☐ Bowel sounds (made by gas and liquid being squeezed around) are heard by listening to the abdomen with a stethoscope. If the bowel stops working, there are no bowel sounds, so silence may be a sign of serious injury. Sometimes, however, bowel sounds may be difficult to hear even in a normal abdomen.

❸ Immediate treatment

IV fluids Fluids will be required if the casualty is shocked. Seek medical advice regarding the type and amount of fluid. Insert an IV cannula (*see* p.172) immediately after assessing the patient, before they become more shocked.

Analgesia Paracetamol, codeine, and even morphine should be used to control the pain. Avoid NSAIDs initially, due to possible complications such as bleeding or bowel perforation.

Antinausea medication Medication should be given to prevent vomiting, which may occur, particularly with severe pain and when using morphine. Seasickness at the time of the accident may compound the problem. The medical kit will contain several different types of antinausea drugs. Medical advice will be useful in deciding which ones to use and in which order (*see* p.147).

Nasogastric (NG) tube An NG tube may be necessary. Abdominal injury can stop the gut from working properly, causing it to fill up with gastric secretions, become distended, and the casualty may then be sick. An NG tube attached to a drainage bag (*see* p.186) will allow the stomach contents to pass up the tube into the bag, reducing the risk of distension, pain, and sickness. Seek medical advice first.

Penetrating wounds Wounds of this type are a serious risk to life: seek medical advice immediately. They should be explored for foreign bodies cautiously and only following medical advice. Protruding foreign bodies should not be removed because they may be plugging a hole in an internal organ or blood vessel. The wound should be cleaned as far as possible, covered with a sterile dressing, and examined and redressed every day until evacuation. Any signs of spreading infection, discharge, or bad smell from the wound suggests infection. Seek medical advice immediately.

Protruding bowel A protruding bowel injury is both serious and distressing. After transferring the casualty to a safe place, cover the bowel with warm, sterile, damp gauze. Seek medical advice immediately.

Antibiotics Any penetrating wound calls for antibiotics, as does any blunt injury if the casualty starts to run a temperature.

❹ Complications

Shock Both blood loss and increasing infection might cause shock. Both situations are very serious, and the casualty will require fluid to make up for the losses. For a shocked casualty, IV fluid is preferred.

Infection An infection may become apparent only in the days following penetrating or blunt injury to the abdomen. It may be a sign that the bowel itself is perforated. Antibiotics should be used for all penetrating injuries and after blunt injuries if the casualty starts to run a temperature or develops signs of peritonitis.

Nausea and vomiting Sickness may start hours or days after the injury and may be a sign of deterioration. Insert an NG tube if one is not already in place and administer antinausea medication through the tube. Examine the abdomen for increasing distension, tenderness, or any masses. The crew should not take anything by mouth.

Blood in the urine Passing blood in the urine may be a sign of injury to one or both kidneys, the tube from the kidney to the bladder (the ureter), the bladder itself, or the tube from the bladder to the outside (the urethra). Offshore, it's not possible to find out exactly where the blood is coming from, but the danger is that it may clot in the bladder, causing the casualty to go into retention (unable to pass urine). Seek medical advice before considering passing a catheter, because this may make matters worse. Continual blood loss over several days may cause the blood pressure to drop and the casualty to become anaemic. Replace fluids and arrange for urgent evacuation.

Hydration and nutrition Both should be maintained, but this may be difficult if the casualty has a distended, painful abdomen and is vomiting; IV fluids may be required. It is possible to give fluids via a rectal tube (*see* p.188), but this is not easy and the absorption rate is limited. The casualty might need more than 3L per day after the initial resuscitation, at which rate the stock of IV fluid on the boat will be quickly exhausted. Other boats nearby might carry further stocks. If so, these should be transferred urgently. Monitoring urine output will give a good idea about the state of hydration and whether more fluid is required. A urinary catheter may be needed: a urine output of about 0.5–1ml per kilogram of body weight per hour should be the aim. Seek medical advice regarding fluid resuscitation and ongoing fluid requirements.

❹ Sites of pain related to organ injuries

This is a general guide relating the site of injury or maximum pain/tenderness to the internal organs that may be damaged. The site of pain may change over time or become generalized if peritonitis develops, so reassess frequently.

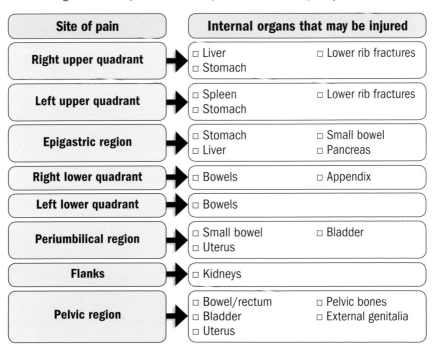

Site of pain	Internal organs that may be injured	
Right upper quadrant	□ Liver □ Stomach	□ Lower rib fractures
Left upper quadrant	□ Spleen □ Stomach	□ Lower rib fractures
Epigastric region	□ Stomach □ Liver	□ Small bowel □ Pancreas
Right lower quadrant	□ Bowels	□ Appendix
Left lower quadrant	□ Bowels	
Periumbilical region	□ Small bowel □ Uterus	□ Bladder
Flanks	□ Kidneys	
Pelvic region	□ Bowel/rectum □ Bladder □ Uterus	□ Pelvic bones □ External genitalia

PELVIC AND HIP INJURIES

Pelvic and hip fractures are usually caused by high energy accidents, such as falls from the rig. Injuries to other parts of the body frequently occur at the same time. Falls from heights greater than 2–3m may also injure the spine.

If the pelvis is fractured, the body's organs in the pelvis may be injured as well (bladder, uterus, urethra, and blood vessels), causing substantial blood loss. The external genitalia may also be injured, and bleeding from the vagina or penis indicates serious injury. In all cases, seek medical advice at an early stage.

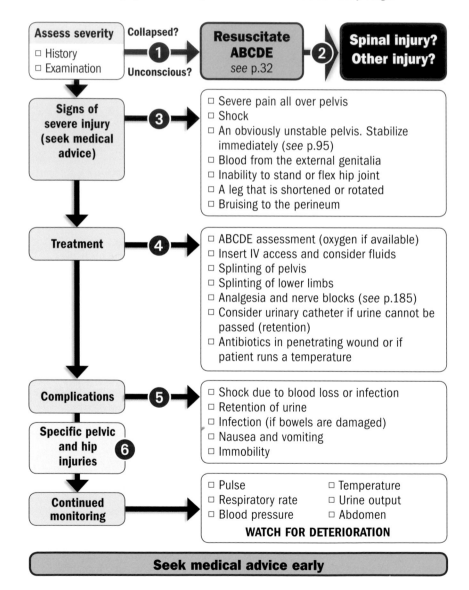

Assess severity
- □ History
- □ Examination

Collapsed? ❶ **Unconscious?**

Resuscitate ABCDE *see p.32*

❷ **Spinal injury? Other injury?**

Signs of severe injury (seek medical advice) ❸
- □ Severe pain all over pelvis
- □ Shock
- □ An obviously unstable pelvis. Stabilize immediately (*see* p.95)
- □ Blood from the external genitalia
- □ Inability to stand or flex hip joint
- □ A leg that is shortened or rotated
- □ Bruising to the perineum

Treatment ❹
- □ ABCDE assessment (oxygen if available)
- □ Insert IV access and consider fluids
- □ Splinting of pelvis
- □ Splinting of lower limbs
- □ Analgesia and nerve blocks (*see* p.185)
- □ Consider urinary catheter if urine cannot be passed (retention)
- □ Antibiotics in penetrating wound or if patient runs a temperature

Complications ❺
- □ Shock due to blood loss or infection
- □ Retention of urine
- □ Infection (if bowels are damaged)
- □ Nausea and vomiting
- □ Immobility

Specific pelvic and hip injuries ❻

Continued monitoring
- □ Pulse
- □ Respiratory rate
- □ Blood pressure
- □ Temperature
- □ Urine output
- □ Abdomen

WATCH FOR DETERIORATION

Seek medical advice early

❶ History and examination

The cause of the accident may indicate the severity of injury. Check for spinal injuries.

Important points in the history

☐ How did the accident happen?
☐ Site and severity of pain?
☐ Can the casualty stand up?
☐ Any blood in the urine?

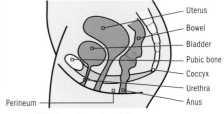

Uterus
Bowel
Bladder
Pubic bone
Coccyx
Urethra
Perineum — Anus

Side view of female pelvic organs

Important points in the examination

Look

☐ Obvious deformity of pelvis
☐ Leg shortened or rotated in or out
☐ Bleeding from vagina or penis
☐ Bruising of perineum

Feel

☐ Use the spring test (*see* below) to look for abnormal movement of pelvis
☐ Rigid, tender abdomen

Listen

☐ Bowel sounds in lower right abdomen

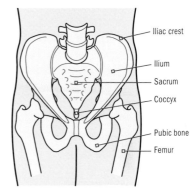

Iliac crest
Ilium
Sacrum
Coccyx
Pubic bone
Femur

Front view of pelvic area

Dealing with an unstable pelvis

A "pelvic spring" test should not be performed. A suspected or obviously unstable pelvis (where it looks deformed) should be stabilized and immobilized immediately. A pelvic binder (either a dedicated one, or one made from equipment on the vessel) should be applied.

❷ Spinal injury

Falls from heights greater than 2–3m may cause spinal injury. The bones of the spine may be broken, but the spinal cord may still be intact. If in doubt, immobilize the casualty on a spinal board (*see* p.165) and check for other injuries.

❸ Signs of severe pelvic or hip injury

☐ A fractured pelvis is usually extremely painful, and the casualty cannot stand.
☐ May result in rapid blood loss of up to 3L, causing life-threatening shock.
☐ Bleeding from the penis or vagina indicates damage to the bladder or urethra, which can be injured when the pelvis is fractured.
☐ With the casualty lying flat, check if one leg is shorter than the other and rotated inwards or outwards. Bending the leg at the hip may cause severe pain. Do this only once as it may cause further bleeding.
☐ Pelvic injury may cause internal bleeding, which shows as "bruising" to the perineum (the area between the top of the legs, behind the scrotum or vagina).

④ Immediate treatment

IV fluids Fluids may be required if the casualty is shocked. Seek medical advice regarding the amount of fluid. Insert an IV cannula immediately after assessing the patient (*see* pp.172–173), before the the shock worsens.

Analgesia Painkillers for moderate to severe pain. Use paracetamol, codeine, tramadol, or morphine to control the pain to a tolerable level. Initially, avoid NSAIDs, which may worsen bleeding. Seek medical advice before using morphine or tramadol.

Nerve blocks Local anaesthetic injections are effective for relieving the pain of hip fractures (*see* p.185). They will last for a few hours and can be repeated.

Splinting of the pelvis Pelvis splinting will reduce blood loss and is relatively simple (*see* illustration below). Doing this as soon as possible will reduce complications.

Splinting of lower limbs Lower limb splinting is useful for both pelvis and hip fractures (*see* illustration below). Bind the knees and ankles together with padding in-between. Keep the patient flat on their back, with a pillow under their knees.

Urinary catheter If a pelvic fracture damages the urethra or the bladder and prevents the casualty from passing urine, a catheter may be required. Seek medical advice before inserting a urinary catheter, as the insertion may cause further damage.

Antibiotics Administer antibiotics for any penetrating wound and also for blunt injuries if the casualty starts to run a temperature.

⑤ Complications

Shock Both blood loss and escalating infection may cause the casualty to go into shock. Both are very serious situations, and the casualty will require fluid. For a shocked casualty, the IV route is preferred.

Retention of urine Blood clots in the bladder or swelling of damaged tissues may result in urine retention over time. Monitor urine output and watch for increasing swelling and pain in the lower abdomen, which may be due to an enlarging bladder. Suprapubic aspiration may be required (*see* p.188).

Infection May develop gradually; may indicate bowel perforation. Use antibiotics for all penetrating injuries and after a blunt injury if casualty starts to run a temperature.

Nausea and vomiting May take hours to develop, indicating injury to the gut. An NG tube should be inserted and antinausea medication given. Look for distension or tenderness in the abdomen. The casualty should take nothing by mouth.

Immobility Initially, the casualty should not move, to reduce the risk of further bleeding, and should be placed in a comfortable position in an accessible bunk and wedged in place to avoid rolling. He or she will still need to pass urine (into a bottle) and may need to open the bowels. A bowl and plastic bag might be used as a makeshift bedpan. If the legs and ankles are splinted together, make sure there is padding in-between, to reduce the risk of pressure sores.

⑥ Specific pelvic and hip injuries

Pelvic fracture

Any part of the pelvis may be fractured, and all types of pelvic fracture involve a risk of severe bleeding. Injury to the spine and to other organs in the region may also be present.

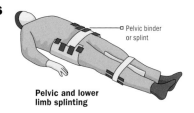

Pelvic binder or splint

Pelvic and lower limb splinting

<table>
<tr><td>

Symptoms and signs

- ☐ Severe pain in the pelvic/lower abdominal area
- ☐ Unable to stand up or flex hip
- ☐ Blood from the vagina or penis
- ☐ Bruised perineum
- ☐ Positive spring test (see p.95)
- ☐ Examine very carefully for other injuries (especially spinal injuries)
- ☐ There may be signs of bowel injury (rigid tender abdomen, possibly becoming distended after hours/days)

</td><td>

Treatment

- ☐ Fluid resuscitation (see pp.170–71)
- ☐ Analgesia and antibiotics
- ☐ Pelvic splinting
- ☐ Lower limb splinting
- ☐ Place in an accessible bunk and wedge in a comfortable position
- ☐ Minimize all movement
- ☐ Pad all bony prominences and area between splinted legs
- ☐ Look for urinary retention; seek advice before inserting a catheter

</td></tr>
</table>

Hip fracture or dislocation

A hip fracture or dislocation requires a lot of force. Other injuries may also be present. A fractured hip usually causes the leg to rotate outwards; a dislocated hip usually causes the leg to rotate inwards. The latter is an emergency. The casualty must be evacuated immediately, or an attempt should be made to relocate the dislocation (see p.194). Seek medical advice before doing so.

<table>
<tr><td>

Symptoms and signs

- ☐ Severe pain from the hip or more generalized over the pelvis
- ☐ Unable to stand or flex hip
- ☐ Inwards- or outwards-rotated leg
- ☐ Possible loss of sensation to leg

</td><td>

Treatment

- ☐ Fluid resuscitation (see pp.170–71)
- ☐ Analgesia
- ☐ If dislocation suspected, seek medical advice before relocating
- ☐ Lower limb splinting (see opposite)

</td></tr>
</table>

Urethral injury

The urethra is the tube by which urine passes from the bladder to the outside. It may be damaged by pelvic fracture, preventing urine from being passed.

<table>
<tr><td>

Symptoms and signs

- ☐ Blood from tip of penis or vagina
- ☐ Blood in the urine
- ☐ Pain passing urine
- ☐ Inability to pass urine
- ☐ Bruising of the perineum/scrotum
- ☐ Full and increasingly painful bladder

</td><td>

Treatment

- ☐ A urinary catheter might be needed, but seek medical advice
- ☐ Suprapubic aspiration might be needed (see p.188)
- ☐ Antibiotics if a urethral or bladder injury is suspected

</td></tr>
</table>

Coccyx injury

Injury to the coccyx can be very painful; on a boat it is impossible to differentiate between bad bruising and a fracture. Bad fractures may result in chronic pain.

<table>
<tr><td>

Symptoms and signs

- ☐ Pain and tenderness over the base of the spine
- ☐ Pain on passing stool

</td><td>

Treatment

- ☐ Analgesia
- ☐ If difficult to pass stool due to pain, use hydration and softening laxatives

</td></tr>
</table>

LIMBS: FRACTURE AND DISLOCATION

Fractures, particularly of the femur, can cause significant blood loss, resulting in shock. Immobilizing a fracture, or putting the ends back together ("reducing" the fracture, see pp.192–93), will reduce pain and limit bleeding. Fractures and dislocations may cause damage to the blood and nerve supply beyond the site of injury, and urgent reduction may be required, following medical advice.

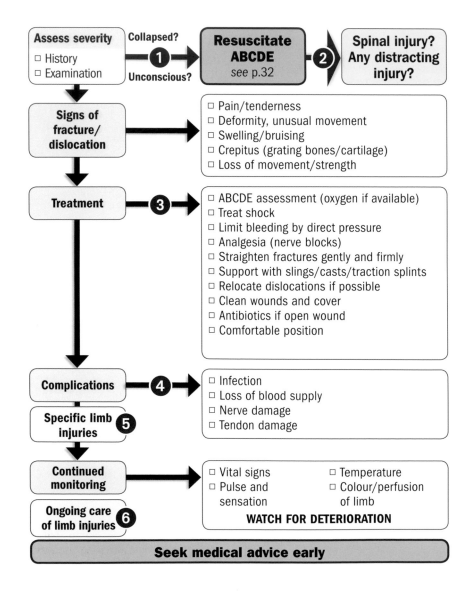

Assess severity
- ☐ History
- ☐ Examination

Collapsed? **1** Unconscious?

Resuscitate ABCDE *see p.32* **2**

Spinal injury? Any distracting injury?

Signs of fracture/ dislocation
- ☐ Pain/tenderness
- ☐ Deformity, unusual movement
- ☐ Swelling/bruising
- ☐ Crepitus (grating bones/cartilage)
- ☐ Loss of movement/strength

Treatment **3**
- ☐ ABCDE assessment (oxygen if available)
- ☐ Treat shock
- ☐ Limit bleeding by direct pressure
- ☐ Analgesia (nerve blocks)
- ☐ Straighten fractures gently and firmly
- ☐ Support with slings/casts/traction splints
- ☐ Relocate dislocations if possible
- ☐ Clean wounds and cover
- ☐ Antibiotics if open wound
- ☐ Comfortable position

Complications **4**
Specific limb injuries **5**
- ☐ Infection
- ☐ Loss of blood supply
- ☐ Nerve damage
- ☐ Tendon damage

Continued monitoring
Ongoing care of limb injuries **6**
- ☐ Vital signs
- ☐ Pulse and sensation
- ☐ Temperature
- ☐ Colour/perfusion of limb

WATCH FOR DETERIORATION

Seek medical advice early

❶ History and examination

- Femoral fractures may be life-threatening due to blood loss
- Upper limb injuries are rarely life threatening
- However, shoulder and collar bone injuries may be associated with spinal injuries
- Painful limb injuries may distract from other more serious injuries

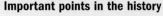

Clavicle
Scapula
Humerus

Ulna
Radius
Pelvis

Femur

Patella

Tibia

Fibula

Common fracture sites

Important points in the history

- How did the accident happen?
- Where and when did it happen?
- Possibility of contamination of wound?
- Any possibility of crushing?
- Any other injuries?
- Any previous fractures or dislocations of the same part?
- Last tetanus injection?

Important points in the examination

Look
- Swelling, bruising
- Deformity
- Open wound over fracture site
- Colour of limb

Feel
- Pain, tenderness
- Bone edges
- Crepitus
- Pulses/perfusion beyond fracture
- Sensation beyond fracture

Move
- Ask the casualty to move the limb first, as far as possible in all directions
- Then move the limb yourself very gently, and stop if causing pain

Document Findings and vital signs

❷ Spinal injury

Distracting injuries may divert attention away from spinal damage. Injuries to the shoulder or clavicle (collar bone) may be very painful and can be associated with fractures of the neck. The force required to break the femur may also cause spinal injuries. The bones of the spine may be broken and unstable, but the spinal cord may still be intact. If in any doubt, immobilize the cervical spine (*see* pp.164–65).

❸ Immediate treatment

Limit bleeding Bleeding may be internal or external and should be limited to avoid shock. Aim to immobilize or reduce the fraction (*see* p.192) as soon as possible. A traction splint (*see* p.189) is effective in stabilizing and reducing a femoral fracture, which may cause heavy blood loss.

Analgesia Fractures are painful, and any attempt at reducing the fracture or dislocation will cause more pain. Analgesia will be needed. Morphine or tramadol may be required, together with antinausea drugs. Nerve blocks may help (*see* p.185).

Reduce fractures Reduce gently, with firm pressure but without force (*see p.192*) as soon as possible – if the surrounding muscles go into spasm, the task will be harder. Analgesia and possibly sedation will be needed to relax the muscles. Reduction is the best way to minimize blood loss and pain. Do not make more than two or three attempts, as each attempt may cause more damage.

Reduce dislocation Shoulder or elbow relocation may be needed, particularly if evacuation will take more than a few hours, because the blood or nerve supply to the arm might be cut off. Before and after attempting relocation, check pulses, colour, and temperature of the arm, and whether the crew can feel your touch.

Clean wounds, cover, give antibiotics This applies to all wounds near a suspected fracture. The bone may have come out through the skin and gone back inside again during the accident, potentially contaminating bone and tissue, or may still be protruding. The bone ends may go back under the skin during reduction. Clean thoroughly, cover with a sterile dressing, and start antibiotics immediately.

Splinting/support Whether or not reduction of the fracture or dislocation has succeeded, splinting or support is needed to reduce pain, bleeding, and swelling.

Keep in a comfortable position Wedged in a bunk is ideal, avoiding pressure on the affected dislocation or fracture.

④ Complications

Infection Inspect wounds regularly for signs of discharge, spreading inflammation, pain, or swelling of the skin. Seek medical advice regarding antibiotic treatment.

Loss of blood supply This may occur immediately or gradually over hours or days. If it does, the limb will not survive very long, and you should seek medical advice urgently. Treat any signs of shock with appropriate fluid, to restore blood pressure to normal (*see pp.166–67*). Elevation of the limb may help reduce swelling, as will prompt reduction of fractures or dislocations. Keep the limb warm.

Nerve damage This may be apparent immediately or may become obvious later. Loss of motor function or sensation may be reversible and may improve over time. On the boat, the best treatments are to promptly reduce any fractures or dislocations (checking nerve function before and after each attempt), treat shock to restore blood pressure, and reduce swelling of the limb by elevation.

Tendon damage This complication cannot be treated on-board. The extent of disability will depend upon which tendons have been damaged, and it may not be possible to flex or extend the limb properly with full power. Thoroughly clean and repair any open wounds, treat with antibiotics, and splint and immobilize the limb to prevent further injury. Evacuation should be arranged urgently.

⑤ Specific upper and lower limb injuries
Types of fracture

In compound ("open") fractures, the bone may not be protruding from the wound when inspected, as the bone ends may have gone back under the skin. Any fracture with a wound near to the fracture site should be considered as compound. Greenstick fractures (in which the bones bends and then partly splinter) happen only in children, who have more flexible bones.

Simple	Compound	Greenstick	Comminuted	Impacted

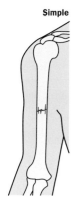 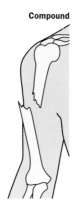 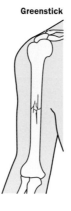 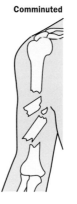 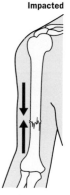

Clavicle fracture and dislocation

The shaft of the clavicle may fracture or the end that connects to the shoulder may dislocate. These injuries may be caused by a direct blow to the shoulder or by a fall onto the shoulder or an outstretched arm. The bone ends might protrude through the skin.

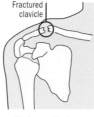

Fractured clavicle

Broken collarbone

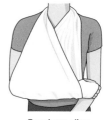

Broad arm sling

Symptoms and signs	Treatment
□ Tenderness over clavicle □ Possible deformity (at the outer end over the shoulder if dislocated) □ Tenting of skin over fractured bone ends □ Reduced and painful shoulder movements	□ Analgesia □ Immobilize and support the arm using a broad arm sling (see above) □ The broken ends of a displaced clavicular fracture may threaten to break the skin. Gentle traction on the arm, pulling away from the center line, may re-oppose the ends, reducing the risk of open fracture.

Shoulder dislocation

Shoulder dislocations are caused by moderate force, such as a fall onto the shoulder or blow to the upper arm. Less force may cause a dislocation if the joint has been dislocated before. The head of the humerus normally dislocates to the front (anteriorly), but may also dislocate downwards (the casualty cannot lower their arm) or backwards (posteriorly) – the upper arm is rotated towards the midline.

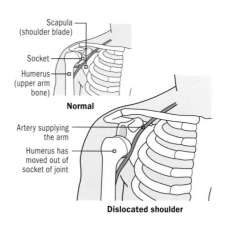

Scapula (shoulder blade)

Socket

Humerus (upper arm bone)

Normal

Artery supplying the arm

Humerus has moved out of socket of joint

Dislocated shoulder

Symptoms and signs	Treatment
□ Severe pain □ Restricted movement of arm □ "Squaring" of shoulder (anterior dislocation) □ Loss of blood or nerve supply to arm (pulses and perfusion of skin) □ Crepitus on movement (a sign of possible fracture-dislocation)	□ Analgesia □ Attempt reduction if blood or nerve supply is reduced (see p.193). Seek medical advice □ Support arm with broad arm sling □ Do not attempt reduction of the fracture if there is crepitus □ Evacuate as soon as possible

Humerus, forearm, and wrist fractures
These injuries are normally caused by falls onto an outstretched hand or onto the elbow. Blood and nerve supply may be compromised.

Symptoms and signs	Treatment
□ Bruising/swelling/deformity □ Loss of movement, crepitus □ Open wounds and bleeding □ Loss of pulses/perfusion/nerve supply to distal limb	□ Analgesia □ Stop bleeding by direct pressure □ Clean/cover open wounds; antibiotics □ Reduce and splint (see pp.193-194) □ Support with a collar and cuff sling

Elbow fracture and dislocation
Dislocation requires considerable force, caused by a direct blow or a fall onto an outstretched hand. It is often combined with a fracture. Blood vessels and nerves to the lower arm all pass close to the elbow joint and may be damaged.

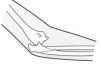

Dislocated elbow

Symptoms and signs	Treatment
□ Pain to elbow and lower arm □ Deformity, loss of movement □ Loss of pulses/perfusion/nerve supply to distal limb	□ Analgesia □ Attempt reduction if blood or nerve supply is reduced (see p.193) □ Support the arm in a broad sling

Femoral fracture
Substantial force is required to fracture the femur, such as that generated by falling from the rig. Other injuries are common. Seek medical advice immediately.

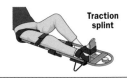

Traction splint

Symptoms and signs	Treatment
□ Severe pain □ Shock □ Deformity of the thigh (one side may appear shortened and thicker) □ Loss of movement □ Inability to stand □ Loss of blood and nerve supply to lower leg	□ Limit external bleeding by immediate immobilization □ Treat shock with fluids □ Analgesia (consider a femoral nerve block – see p.185) □ Apply traction splint (see p.189) □ Treat open wounds (antibiotics) □ Seek medical advice and evacuate

Knee injuries

Knees are prone to injury on boats, and occasionally the patella (kneecap) may be become dislocated laterally (away from the midline) or even fractured by a direct blow or sudden flexion. If there is immediate significant swelling and deformity, fracture of the distal femur and dislocation of the knee are possibilities (both require major force). If in any doubt, seek medical advice. For ligament injuries, see also pp.108–110.

Symptoms and signs	Treatment

□ Pain
□ Swelling around knee
□ Inability to perform straight leg raise
□ Patella dislocation
  – Deformity on lateral side of knee
  – Leg held in slight flexion
	□ Analgesia
	□ Suspected patella fracture
	  – Immobilize with the knee slightly bent, using a full leg splint
	  – Evacuate urgently
	□ Suspected patella dislocation
	  – Relocate the patella by straightening the leg and pushing the patella back in place firmly with thumbs
	  – Support the knee with crepe or elastic support bandage

Lower leg fractures

Fracture of the tibia is relatively common on boats. High-energy accidents, such as falls from the rig or down the companionway or being swept down the deck, may cause a displaced fracture, which can be open. Badly displaced fractures may cause significant swelling of the lower leg, cutting off blood and nerve supply to the distal limb. Urgent evacuation is required in such cases.

Symptoms and signs	Treatment
□ Pain at site of fracture □ Deformity □ Swelling (the calf may become very tense over a few hours or days) □ Crepitus □ Loss of distal perfusion and pulses □ Reduced distal sensation □ Inability to bear weight	□ Analgesia □ Stop bleeding by direct pressure □ Clean and cover wounds □ Reduce fracture and splint – a traction splint may be effective (see p.189) □ Antibiotics for open fracture □ Elevate leg to reduce swelling □ Evacuate urgently if open displaced fracture or significant swelling

⑥ Ongoing care of fractures and dislocations

□ Keep the casualty comfortably wedged in a bunk, where you can more easily examine the wounds.
□ Use analgesia to control the pain – more if the casualty is being moved.
□ Elevate the injured limb as much as possible.
□ Watch for limb swelling and distal perfusion (see p.167).
□ Encourage the casualty to mobilize as soon as possible, as pain allows.

HAND, FOOT, AND ANKLE INJURIES

Appropriate gloves and shoes afford some protection from hand and foot injuries, which are common on boats. The most frequent injuries are rope burns, finger dislocation, crushing, and skin loss. Deep lacerations heal poorly and often need suturing.

History and examination

Remove rings and bracelets immediately, before swelling occurs. Note that injury to the dominant hand is disabling.

Important points in the history

- ☐ How did the accident happen?
- ☐ Where and when did it happen?
- ☐ Possibility of contamination of wound?
- ☐ Any possibility of crushing?
- ☐ Other injuries?
- ☐ Previous fractures or dislocations of the same part?
- ☐ Last tetanus injection?

Important points in the examination

Look
- ☐ Swelling; bruising; deformity
- ☐ Open wound over fracture site
- ☐ Colour of toes (with ankle injury)

Feel
- ☐ Pain, tenderness
- ☐ Bone edges
- ☐ Crepitus (bone grating)
- ☐ Perfusion beyond fracture
- ☐ Sensation beyond fracture

Move
- ☐ Casualty to check limits of movement
- ☐ Move the hand or foot gently yourself

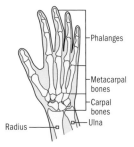

Bones of the hand

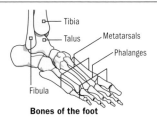

Bones of the foot

Immediate treatment

Stop bleeding Apply direct pressure or a blood pressure cuff around the forearm or lower leg. After the hand or foot has been inspected, elevated, and dressed, remove pressure cuff immediately or there may be damage caused by lack of blood supply.

Analgesia Consider ring blocks and infiltration for pain relief (see pp.184–85).

Clean wounds, cover, and give antibiotics Inspect all wounds for foreign bodies and damage to underlying bones, tendons, and nerves.

Reduce or relocate fractures and dislocations See pp.192–195.

Support and elevate Compression bandage, splint, elevation to reduce swelling.

Specific injuries

Hand and foot fractures and crush injuries

Serious hand and foot injuries may require urgent evacuation to avoid loss of vital function. Seek medical advice if in any doubt regarding severity of injury.

High arm sling

Symptoms and signs	Specific treatment
□ Deformity, swelling, bruising □ Pain/tenderness/loss of sensation □ Loss of function (strength, movement)	□ Support arm with high arm sling □ Elevate leg and foot □ Splint if necessary

Finger and toe dislocations and fractures

These wounds are often caused by the finger being forced backwards or the toe stubbed. Buddy splinting to adjacent finger or toe is usually sufficient immobilization.

Dislocated finger   **Buddy splint**

Symptoms and signs	Specific treatment
□ Deformity □ Swelling, bruising □ Loss of function	□ Reduce dislocation and displaced fracture (see p.194) □ Buddy splint (see above)

Finger and toe crush injuries and de-gloving

Finger and toe injuries are common on boats, especially in the cold, when dexterity and sensation are reduced. Seek medical advice in cases of major tissue loss or amputation.

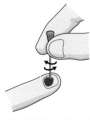

Pierce the nail with a hot, blunt needle to drain a haematoma. A fine drill bit can also be used, with the fingers, to "drill" a small hole.

Symptoms and signs	Specific treatment
□ Deformity, bruising, and swelling □ Skin loss, exposed bone. In skin loss, look for the missing skin □ Pain, blood under nail □ Possible tissue loss	□ In skin loss, cover with damp, sterile dressing and seek medical advice □ Gently pierce nail with a hot pin, to relieve pressure of blood under nail

Ankle fracture or dislocation

Fractures of the ankle are relatively common. Dislocations are less common; they are serious and require urgent evacuation.

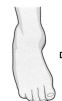

Dislocated ankle

Symptoms and signs	Specific treatment
□ Ankle deformity, worse in dislocation □ Swelling, bruising □ Loss of function □ Severe deformity may cause loss of blood and nerve supply to foot	□ Reduce dislocation urgently if nerve and blood supply are reduced (see p.195) □ Compression dressings and supportive splint (see pp.189-90) □ Elevate leg and foot □ Arrange urgent evacuation

FISH HOOK INJURIES

Injuries involving fish hooks are all too common. Prevention is by far the best approach, so the use of gloves while fishing is thoroughly recommended. Fish hooks are a potent source of infection, which may complicate injuries.

Fish hooks can become embedded in exposed skin anywhere on the body, but the usual sites are the hands, the feet, and occasionally the head, including lips, ears, and eyes. Penetrating eye injuries are serious; you should seek medical advice and arrange urgent evacuation. Fortunately, hooks usually become embedded at a shallow depth, parallel with the skin surface, because of the way they are designed.

A range of fish hooks are illustrated opposite. They demonstrate the problem with removing an embedded fish hook: hooks are usually barbed, with one point barb normally but occasionally with multiple barbs, which prevent easy extraction. There are various methods of removing a fish hook. Knowing the type of hook before attempting extraction is an advantage.

Some methods of extraction cause further injury by pushing the hook through the skin and out again. Additional trauma is, of course, painful and generally not desirable. However, these methods tend to have a higher rate of success. The other methods described here involve extracting the hook back along the route of entry. This causes less pain and trauma, but tends to be less successful.

Fish hook removal

Initial preparation
☐ Remove line, lures, and tackle.
☐ Remove extra points on the same hook.
☐ Clean the skin with topical antiseptic (applied directly to the skin).
☐ Local anaesthetic or freezing spray; nerve block for fingers or toes (see p.185).
☐ Treat hooks embedded in the eye with antibiotic drops. Seek medical advice and evacuate urgently.

Method 1: Push forwards and cut
☐ Push the hook onwards, angling the shank to ensure that the point and barb come out through the skin.
☐ This is painful, so administer local anaesthetic.
☐ Cut the point and barb off and pull backwards, or cut off the hook eye and continue to pull through, if the shank is barbed (see diagram).
☐ A pair of pliers is the ideal tool.

Advantage   Usually successful
Disadvantage   Causes more trauma

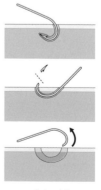

Cut point and barb

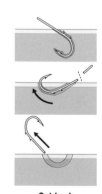

Cut hook eye

Types of fish hook	Hook anatomy

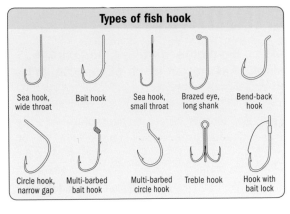

Sea hook, wide throat   Bait hook   Sea hook, small throat   Brazed eye, long shank   Bend-back hook

Circle hook, narrow gap   Multi-barbed bait hook   Multi-barbed circle hook   Treble hook   Hook with bait lock

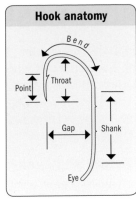

Method 2: Line and pull back

☐ Place a length of line around the bend of the hook.
☐ Press down over the point and barb to attempt to disengage the barb from the tissue.
☐ Pull back on the line firmly along the line of the shank, which should be held down to ensure that the point and barb exit the skin (see diagram).
☐ Dispose of the extracted hook safely.

Advantage   Quite successful
Disadvantage   Hook comes out at some rate and causes pain

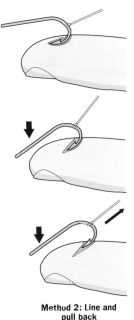

Method 2: Line and pull back

Method 3: Straight reverse extraction

☐ Push down on the shank to rotate the point and barb deeper, aiming to disengage the barb from the skin (see diagram).
☐ Gently work the hook out backwards along the line of entry.
☐ Patience may be needed to gradually extract the needle without the barb becoming caught.

Advantage   A simple technique, causing little further injury
Disadvantage   A low success rate

Aftercare Allow the wound to bleed, then clean, dress, and elevate. Treat with antibiotics and analgesia. Watch for spreading infection (redness, swelling, and pain around wounds) and check tetanus status.

Complications There is a risk of infection, both of the site and the underlying structures (nerves, tendons, and blood vessels, which may also be damaged in the initial injury). Retained foreign bodies may necessitate X-ray and surgical exploration.

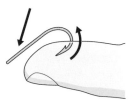

Method 3: Straight reverse extraction

SOFT TISSUE INJURIES

Injuries to muscles, tendons, ligaments, cartilage, and bursae go hand in hand with sailing, and are the result of impacts, falls, twists, heavy lifting, and repetitive overuse.

The principles of treatment are the same for most injuries. Be aware of the risks, use protective clothing, and make sure injuries are recognized and treated early.

History and examination

- The injury may be acute (caused by an accident) or chronic (repetitive action)
- Inflammation and infection may complicate injury and need treatment
- The injured part is at risk of further injury
- If in any doubt, treat it as a fracture
- Further investigation may be required

Important points in the history

- When, where, how did it happen?
- Sudden or gradual onset?
- Site and severity of pain?
- Previous similar injuries?

Definitions

Ligament A fibrous rope connecting bones or cartilage, serving to support and strengthen joints
Tendon A fibrous rope attaching the muscle to bone or cartilage
Cartilage A piece of fibrous tissue that forms part of the flexible skeleton
Bursa A fluid-filled lubricating sac situated in places in tissues where friction would otherwise occur.

Important points in the examination

Look
- Deformity
- Swelling, bruising
- Redness

Feel
- Site of tenderness
- Feel for fluid around joint
- Bone grating if possible fracture
- Warmth of joint (may be infected)

Move
- Ask the casualty to move the injured part, as far as possible, in all directions, testing strength
- Then move the injured part yourself, very gently, stopping if causing pain

Document Findings such as range of movement and what elicits pain

Signs of severe injury

- Severe pain
- Immediate swelling
- Total loss of movement
- Obvious bruising

Immediate treatment

Painkillers NSAIDs provide effective pain relief and reduce inflammation. However, if there is severe bruising, avoid NSAIDs for the first 24 hours, as they may worsen bleeding. Morphine or tramadol is rarely required. Extreme pain usually indicates a more severe injury, such as a fracture.

Rest Rest for 24–72 hours, depending on severity. If this is not possible, immobilize and support the affected joint by taping or splinting (see pp.189–90).

Ice Apply ice immediately to reduce swelling and speed recovery. Avoid direct contact with the skin, as this may cause a cold injury. Apply the pack for 15 minutes 4–6 times a day for 48 hours, longer if having to mobilize with protection/support straight after the injury. Alternatives to ice include cold aerosol spray, a cold pack, or a cloth soaked in cold water.

Compression Use a crepe bandage or elasticated tubular support bandage, especially when mobilizing (correct size to avoid excess compression and reduced blood flow – check distal limb perfusion). This will help to support the injury, reduce further damage, and remind the casualty to protect the injured part.

Elevation Raising the limb will also reduce swelling. An injured arm should be held above the heart in a high arm sling (*see* p.191) and an injured leg should be elevated with the foot higher than the hip. Maintain elevation as much as possible.

Mobilization Moving the injured joint or muscle aids recovery, as long as it is controlled. If mobilizing immediately after injury, protect the injured part with splinting or taping and compression. When mobilizing after 24–72 hours, use compression dressing, elevate when resting, and resume use gradually.

Specific injuries

Grazes, bruises, rope burns

Symptoms and signs	Treatment
□ Very common, usually acutely painful □ Potentially contaminated □ Large bruises (haematomas) may become infected and form abscesses	□ Clean thoroughly, remove foreign bodies, and apply sterile dressing □ Antibiotic cream/ointment/oral □ Abscesses may need incision and drainage (*see* p.183)

Shoulder injuries

Excessive strain can damage the shoulder muscles (rotator cuff). Tasks that require repetitive actions such as helming and sail trimming can inflame tendons and bursae.

Symptoms and signs	Treatment
□ Restricted movement □ Pain on movement □ Sudden onset is usually a strain or muscle tear □ Tendonitis/bursitis usually gradual	□ Rest – immobilization in severe cases (broad arm sling) □ NSAIDs □ Gradual return to activity □ Change method of activity

Elbow and wrist injures

These joints are prone to repetitive strain injury ("wincher's elbow"), which causes tenosynovitis. Trauma to the point of the elbow may cause bursitis.

Symptoms and signs	Treatment
□ Restricted movement □ Pain on movement and making a fist □ Swelling over the elbow (bursitis), which feels soft and unstable. Swelling might be tight and painful □ Infection – redness, swelling, warmth	□ Rest and wrist splinting □ Strap around forearm muscles for winchers elbow (not too tight) □ Tight fluid swelling: aspirate with needle/syringe. Seek medical advice □ Antibiotics for signs of infection

Knee injuries

The ligaments, bursae, tendons, and cartilage in the knee all serve to stabilize the joint. Any and all can be damaged. Knee injuries may be disabling for weeks and may require evacuation. Repeated kneeling often causes bursitis in front of the knee cap.

Symptoms and signs	Treatment
□ Swelling (the knee may swell rapidly and considerably with severe injury) □ Restricted, painful movement □ Instability on weight bearing is a sign of ligament injury □ "Locking" of the knee on movement is a sign of cartilage damage inside the knee □ Infection – redness, warmth over knee	□ Rest, ice, compression, elevation □ Pain relief (NSAIDs) □ Immobilization (splinting) for serious injury – evacuate □ Aspirate tense swellings with needle and syringe. Seek medical advice first □ Antibiotics for signs of infection □ Careful mobilization as tolerated

Ankle injuries

Injured ankles tend to loose their stability, so take care when mobilizing. It is difficult to tell the difference between a fracture and sprain. On a boat, both are treated in the same way. The large Achilles tendon is at the back of the ankle and can be torn or ruptured by a sudden load on the ankle (for example, jumping down onto the dock). This type of injury is disabling.

Symptoms and signs	Treatment
□ Swelling, bruising □ Pain on movement □ A gap in the Achilles tendon which you may be able to feel □ Tenderness over the ankle bones (medial and lateral malleoli)	□ Rest, ice, compression (strapping), elevation □ Pain relief (NSAIDs) □ For suspected Achilles tendon injury, splint ankle and seek medical advice □ Careful mobilization (possible instability)

Lower back pain

Backs and boats do not go well together, and new exercise may injure the back: muscles, ligaments, intervertebral discs, and nerves may be involved. Rarely, a back injury may be serious and require evacuation. If in any doubt, seek medical advice.

Symptoms and signs	Treatment
□ What movements make the pain worse or better? □ Where is the pain felt: locally in the back, in the legs, one side or both? □ Previous back problems? **Nerve problems** □ Problems with passing water/faeces? □ Burning pain, numbness, or tingling felt in the legs?	□ Rest, but encourage early, careful, gentle mobilization □ Care with activities (no heavy lifting, keep back straight) □ Pain relief (NSAIDs) □ Use of low-dose benzodiazepine (diazepam 1-5mg) may help □ If signs of nerve problems, seek medical advice and evacuate

TREATING PAIN

There is no absolute measure of pain, so the casualty's opinion about the pain they are suffering is the main guide to treatment. If the casualty says they are in pain, believe them.

Treatment of pain is of paramount importance. Pain demoralizes, demotivates, and causes physical stress to the casualty. Controlling pain promotes physical and emotional recovery, enables sleep and mobility, reduces complications, and speeds healing.

Causes of pain

- Obvious wound
- Swelling
- Organ infection or damage
- Fractures
- Abscess
- Lack of blood flow to organ (such as the heart)
- Infection
- Nerve damage
- Increased sensitivity (previous nerve damage)

Signs

Usually the casualty will be able to say whether they are in pain, but sometimes they may not be able to because of confusion, loss of speech, or loss of consciousness. In these cases, there are signs that indicate the existence and severity of pain.

- Grimacing
- Cold to touch
- Pain localizing to a point
- Writhing
- Pale
- Raised heart rate
- Confusion
- Sweating
- Raised breathing rate
- Agitation
- Nausea, vomiting
- Increased depth of breathing

Treatment

Immediate control of pain is the first objective, followed by longer-term measures to reduce pain to a bearable level while healing takes place or evacuation is arranged.

Medications Morphine or tramadol injected intramuscularly provides rapid pain control but may cause nausea, so give an antinausea drug at the same time. For longer term pain relief, use regular paracetamol and NSAIDs (see Pain Ladder, p.212). These will help to avoid the need for morphine or tramadol, which causes sickness, constipation, and drowsiness, and should be kept for emergency use.

Local anaesthesia May be used to numb nerves and reduce pain. Particularly useful for femoral fractures, finger blocks, and repairing wounds (see pp.184–185).

Splintage Immobilizes fractures and reduces bone movement, lessening pain.

Reduction Reducing fractures and dislocations will decrease the likelihood of bleeding, swelling, and nerve damage.

Elevation Raising an injured limb reduces swelling and pain and allows early mobilization.

Cool Sprains and muscle injuries can be cooled to reduce swelling and pain. The same applies to burns.

Warmth/heat Eases muscle discomfort in the days following injury. Take care not to cause burns. On a boat, use a hot water bottle wrapped in a towel or a hot compress.

Dressings Applying dressings to wounds will reduce pain caused by contact.

Medical
Disorders

NEUROLOGICAL DISORDERS

When something goes wrong with all or part of the brain, it may result in loss of consciousness, paralysis, fitting, headache, or changes in behaviour. Some neurological disorders begin spontaneously, in the absence of trauma.

The brain may be affected by various disorders including: bleeding in and around the brain; infection of the brain or the surrounding membranes (the meninges); blood clots, which may reduce blood supply; low blood pressure; low blood glucose; and lack of oxygen. Epilepsy, migraine, and fainting may occur without any obvious brain abnormality.

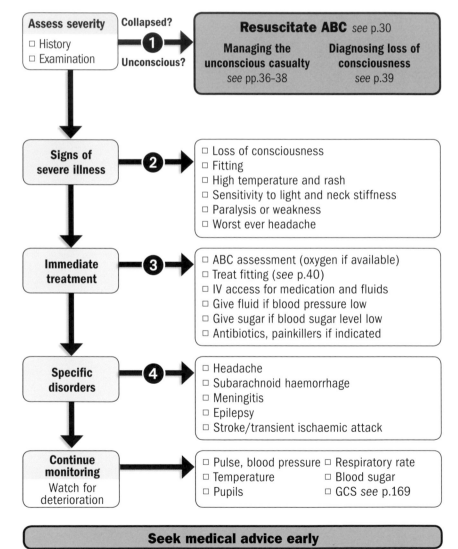

Assess severity
- □ History
- □ Examination

Collapsed?

1

Unconscious?

Resuscitate ABC *see p.30*

Managing the unconscious casualty *see pp.36–38*

Diagnosing loss of consciousness *see p.39*

Signs of severe illness

2

- □ Loss of consciousness
- □ Fitting
- □ High temperature and rash
- □ Sensitivity to light and neck stiffness
- □ Paralysis or weakness
- □ Worst ever headache

Immediate treatment

3

- □ ABC assessment (oxygen if available)
- □ Treat fitting (*see p.40*)
- □ IV access for medication and fluids
- □ Give fluid if blood pressure low
- □ Give sugar if blood sugar level low
- □ Antibiotics, painkillers if indicated

Specific disorders

4

- □ Headache
- □ Subarachnoid haemorrhage
- □ Meningitis
- □ Epilepsy
- □ Stroke/transient ischaemic attack

Continue monitoring
Watch for deterioration

- □ Pulse, blood pressure
- □ Temperature
- □ Pupils
- □ Respiratory rate
- □ Blood sugar
- □ GCS *see p.169*

Seek medical advice early

❶ History and examination

□ It may not be possible to communicate with a casualty who is confused.
□ Use other sources of information – crewmates, initial crew medical questionnaire, next-of-kin over the radio or satellite telephone, medic alert bracelets.
□ Symptoms may take some time to develop, so re-examine regularly.

Important points in the history

□ Did the symptoms start suddenly or did they develop over a few days?
□ Has this happened before?
□ Loss of consciousness?
□ Fitting (generalized/local)?
□ Worst ever headache?
□ Any neck stiffness?
□ Pain when looking at bright light?
□ Any rashes on the body?
□ Weakness in arms/legs
□ Does the casualty take aspirin, clopidogrel, warfarin?

Important points in the examination

Look
□ Obvious signs of illness – pallor, fitting, rashes anywhere on body?
□ Pupil size and reaction to light
□ Oriented in time/place?

Move
□ Ask the casualty to move the arms/legs. Is there weakness, paralysis?
□ Move the limbs gently yourself, looking for stiffness, flaccidity
□ Flex head forwards gently, touching chin to chest; stop if it hurts

---

❷ Signs of severe illness

Loss of consciousness The priority is ABC assessment. *See* pp.41–43 for causes and treatment.

Fitting If fitting carries on for more than 5 minutes, it must be treated. *See* p.40 for causes and treatment.

High temperature and rash A temperature and rash are signs of infection. The rash does not "blanch" when firmly pressed.

Photophobia The casualty will have pain looking into a bright light.

Neck stiffness The casualty will have intense neck pain trying to put chin to chest.

Paralysis or weakness Paralysis down one side of the body – legs or arms may be involved, or one side of the face – may be a sign of a stroke or haemorrhage.

Headache A very severe headache may be caused by a subarachnoid haemorrhage, meningitis, or a stroke (*see* below).

❸ Immediate treatment

Analgesia Pain relief may be required for severe headaches. Use paracetamol and codeine as required, but avoid morphine if possible. NSAIDs may be useful, but do not use them if a bleed in the head is suspected, as they may exacerbate bleeding. Use antinausea medication if required and when using codeine.

Blood sugar Correct blood sugar levels if either very low or very high (*see* p.59).

Antibiotics Give intravenously as a preference, when there are signs of infection and if there is a possibility of meningitis (*see* below).

Fluids Extra fluids may be needed if the casualty has low blood pressure, but excess fluids may not be beneficial for certain disorders. Seek medical advice to guide fluid resuscitation and further hydration.

④ Specific condtions

Headache

Headaches are very common and not usually a problem, but severe or persistent headaches (lasting longer than 24 hours despite treatment with plenty of fluids, simple painkillers, and rest) should be taken seriously.

CAUSES OF HEADACHE	
SERIOUS BUT RARE CAUSES	
Meningitis ┈┈┈┈┈┈┈➤	See opposite page
Subarachnoid haemorrhage ┈┈┈┈➤	See opposite page
Carbon monoxide poisoning ┈┈┈➤	See p.154

LESS SERIOUS, MORE COMMON CAUSES	
Symptoms and signs	**Treatment**
Tension/Tiredness □ General headache and sore neck □ Lack of sleep □ Dehydration	□ Efficient rest □ Good hydration □ Change of helming/trimming position □ Analgesia
Dehydration □ Thirst □ Lethargy, fatigue □ Small amount of dark urine □ Heavy work, sweating □ Tropical climate	□ Attention to drinking plenty of rehydration fluids, especially in hot climates and when working hard □ Work as a team to keep hydrated □ Watch colour of urine – if it goes dark, drink more rehydration fluid
Sinusitis □ Tender over cheek or eyebrow □ Fever □ Foul discharge from nose or back of throat	□ Antibiotics □ Analgesia □ Avoid blowing nose □ Steam inhalation may help □ No diving or air travel
Migraine □ Previous history of migraine? □ Pain is usually on one side of head □ Visual disturbances (blurring, flashing lights, even blindness)	□ Analgesia □ Rest in quiet and dark □ Keep hydrated □ Antinausea medication if sick □ Avoid chocolate, citrus fruits, cheese
Sunstroke □ History of sun exposure without proper protection □ Heavy work in direct sun □ Reddened, painful, itchy skin, blistering	□ Keep out of sun □ Wear sunscreen, hat, shirt □ Cool down (damp clothes, hat) □ Analgesia □ Keep hydrated □ Antinausea medication if sick
Alcohol/drugs □ History of heavy alcohol intake □ Nitrates (glyceryl trinitrate spray) □ Dehydration	□ Avoid certain prescription drugs if they are possibly the cause – seek medical advice □ Moderate alcohol intake

Subarachnoid haemorrhage (SAH)

SAH is the result of a ruptured blood vessel in the head, causing bleeding and pain. It is life-threatening and may result in sudden loss of consciousness.

Symptoms and signs	Treatment
□ Sudden onset worst ever headache – like a blow to the back of head □ Confusion, drowsiness □ Neck pain, vomiting □ Fitting/loss of consciousness	□ Assess ABC (see p.30), oxygen □ Treat fitting (see p.40) □ Analgesia and rest □ Seek medical advice □ Urgent evacuation

Meningitis

When infection causes inflammation of the membrane covering the brain, it is known as meningitis. This condition is life-threatening if not recognized and treated rapidly using antibiotics. Immunization is available and should be considered before voyages.

Symptoms and signs	Treatment
□ Fever and headache for several hours □ Stiff neck □ Photophobia □ Possibly a nonblanching rash □ Later – unconsciousness, shock	□ Assess ABC (see p.30), vital signs □ Antibiotics (preferably IV) □ Analgesia for headache, sore neck □ Seek medical advice □ Urgent evacuation

Epilepsy (for control of fitting – see p.40)

The casualty may be known to suffer from epilepsy and may take medication, but seasickness may prevent oral medication from being absorbed, resulting in fitting. The casualty will be sleepy after the fit (the "post-ictal" period – see p.40).

Symptoms and signs	Treatment
□ Generalized or localized fitting □ Incontinence, tongue biting □ Causes: – Non-absorption of normal meds – Infection – Alcohol withdrawal	□ Assess ABC (see p.30), oxygen □ Prevent injury but do not restrain □ Recovery position □ Treat fitting (see p.40) □ Seek medical advice □ Urgent evacuation

Stroke and transient ischaemic attack (TIA)

A stroke may be caused by a bleed or a blood clot in the brain. A blood clot can also cause a TIA, which may have similar symptoms to a stroke, but symptoms should resolve in an hour or so. Both may be life-threatening events.

Symptoms and signs	Treatment
□ Paralysis down one side of the body, one limb, or side of face □ Difficulty speaking and swallowing □ Visual problems □ Altered sensation/poor coordination □ Headache and possible fitting	□ Assess ABC (see p.30), oxygen □ Treat fitting (see p.40) □ Recovery position if unconscious □ Analgesia if required □ Seek medical advice □ Urgent evacuation

EYE DISORDERS

The eye is relatively well protected within its socket and behind the eyelid, so serious disorders are relatively rare. However, the environment does cause significant problems: wind, snow, UV glare, fatigue, and lack of hygiene all affect the eye, particularly in crew who wear contact lenses or glasses.

Only a few treatments for eye disorders are practical on a boat, such as antibiotic drops or ointment, anaesthetic drops, eye lubrication, rest, and protection, but these measures are effective for most complaints. Some symptoms, such as blindness and a painful red eye, warrant immediate medical advice and urgent evacuation.

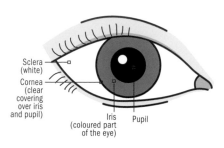

Front view of the eye

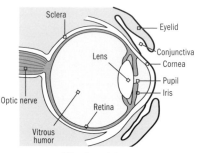

Side view of the eye

History and examination

- ☐ The casualty may have a history of eye problems, which should give you some idea of the diagnosis.
- ☐ Examination needs to be done in a safe and stable place (such as a bunk or saloon), and the area should be well lit (for example, with a head torch).
- ☐ Compare eyes to see if the problem affects both sides.

Important points in the history

- ☐ How quickly have the symptoms developed?
- ☐ Pain? Worse with light?
- ☐ Blurred, poor, or double vision?
- ☐ Any discharge from eye (stickiness)?
- ☐ Previous problems with eyes/vision?
- ☐ Eye surgery in past (cataract/laser)?
- ☐ Contact lenses or glasses?
- ☐ Diabetes, glaucoma, arthritis?
- ☐ Medications for eyes?

Important points in the examination

Look (compare sides)
- ☐ Redness over sclera, discharge?
- ☐ Swellings around eye and lids?
- ☐ Size and reactivity of pupil?
- ☐ Blood or pus in front of the iris?
- ☐ Cloudiness of cornea or lens (pupil should appear clear black)
- ☐ Look inside eyelids (see pp.82–83)

Feel (compare sides)
- ☐ Press gently on globe of eye – painful or very tense?
- ☐ Tenderness around orbit, eyelids?

Move
- ☐ Ask casualty to look at your finger held 30cm away. Move finger up/down and side to side slowly. Keep head still. Ask about double vision and watch eye movements closely.
- ☐ Record which movements cause pain

Visual acuity
- ☐ Test vision by reading small text from a book at normal distance

Using fluorescein drops to help examination of the eye
- □ Fluorescein dye stains abrasion and ulceration of the cornea a greenish colour when lit by blue light.
- □ Put a few drops of tetracaine 0.5% local anaesthetic inside the lower eyelid (fluorescein dye will sting).
- □ After two minutes, put in a few drops of fluorescein inside the lower eyelid.
- □ Close the eye for a minute or so and wipe off excess fluorescein.
- □ Examine the cornea with a magnifying glass and bright light (blue if available).
- □ Stain the eyes one at a time, 30 mins apart.

Signs of severe eye disorders

Blindness: either in one eye or both; may or may not be painful
Reduction in visual acuity: the crew has blurred vision
Red eye: particularly when the eye itself is painful (*see* below)
Unreactive pupil: when a bright light is shone into the eye
Cloudy cornea or lens: the pupil should be clear black

Seek medical advice

Causes of "red eye"

Serious
- □ Acute glaucoma – blurred vision, painful eye
- □ Acute iritis – blurred vision, pain, photophobia
- □ Corneal inflammation/ulceration (keratitis)
- □ Orbital cellulitis – swelling and redness around the eye
- □ Trauma to the eye (*see* pp.84–85)

Seek medical advice

Less serious
- □ Prolonged contact lens use
- □ Conjunctivitis/scleritis
- □ Sea blindness
- □ Subconjunctival haemorrhage
- □ Foreign body in the eye (*see* p.84)

Specific conditions

Contact lens problems
The environment on a boat is not suited to contact lenses. They are more difficult to clean, disposable contacts will be more difficult to replace, and all types will suffer from being exposed to sea, sun, wind, and salt.
- □ Lens stuck in eye: wash out with copious sterile normal saline; someone may need to help by extracting the lens gently.
- □ Sore, dry eyes: *see* p.120
- □ Conjunctivitis: stop wearing the lenses until infection completely clears; sterilize lenses.
- □ Corneal abrasion: a problem with prolonged use. Stop wearing lenses; for treatment, *see* p.84
- □ Lost lens: may still be in the eye but difficult to see. Inspect the inside of the lids thoroughly, particularly the upper lid (*see* p.83).

Dry eyes

Dry eyes result from exposure to sea, sun, salt, and wind. Contact wearers are particularly at risk.

Symptoms and signs	Treatment
□ Eyes are red, painful, and feel gritty □ Both eyes usually affected □ Long period of wearing contact lens	□ Use artificial tears (such as hypromellose) □ Reduce time wearing contact lenses □ Sunglasses/goggles to protect eyes □ Antibiotic ointment may lubricate the eyes and help to relieve pain

Sea blindness ("Sailor's Eye")

This condition is similar to snow blindness or corneal flash burns. It is caused by sunburn of the eye by UV rays and is a particular risk at sea due to surface reflection.

Symptoms and signs	Treatment
□ May happen after only 2-3 hours of exposure □ Very painful red eyes □ Face may be burnt red as well □ Bright light may hurt eye □ Headache is common □ Usually both eyes affected	□ Prevention is best – sunglasses with good protection from the sides □ Assess for foreign bodies first □ Local anaesthetic drops for pain, and oral painkillers for headache □ Antibiotic ointment may lubricate the eyes and help to relieve pain

Conjunctivitis

Conjunctivitis is a serious problem on boats because the whole crew may catch it. Do not share towels or bedding. One eye may be affected, but usually both are.

Symptoms and signs	Treatment
□ Red, painful eye (cornea is not red) □ Discharge of pus – bacterial infection □ Watery discharge – viral infection □ Itchy eye – allergic cause □ Vision not affected	□ Antibiotic drops or ointment for 5 days □ Viral conjunctivitis will clear without treatment □ Antihistamine eye drops if allergic cause suspected

Corneal inflammation/ulceration (keratitis)

Keratitis may cause scarring, which can permanently affect vision. Causes include infection, contact lens overuse, and corneal abrasion. Do not use steroid drops if there is any possibility of corneal infection – this may worsen inflammation.

Symptoms and signs	Treatment
□ Red and painful eye □ Photophobia □ Watering □ Cloudy cornea with bacterial infection □ Blurred vision	□ Ulcers will glow greenish with fluorescein staining □ Antibiotic drops or ointment □ Seek medical advice as vision may be threatened

Subconjunctival haemorrhage

Symptoms and signs	Treatment
□ One eye may appear alarmingly red □ Vision unaffected □ No apparent cause (minor trauma, use of drugs such as aspirin, warfarin)	□ No specific treatment required □ Should clear in 2–3 weeks □ If recurrent, check blood pressure and review medications

Orbital cellulitis

Inflammation of the orbit within which the eye sits is a threat to eyesight. IV antibiotics should be used.

Symptoms and signs	Treatment
□ Painful, red eye □ Swelling around eye, possibly causing lids to close □ Possible loss of vision □ Fever and feeling unwell	□ IV antibiotics □ Hydration □ Analgesia as required □ Seek medical advice immediately □ Arrange urgent evacuation

Acute glaucoma

A build-up of fluid pressure within the eye may threaten sight. Usually, only one eye is affected. Pilocarpine 0.5% drops may be available for emergency treatment.

Symptoms and signs	Treatment
□ Pain, nausea, vomiting □ Red eye around the cornea, which might be hazy □ Blurred vision, halos □ Semi-dilated/unresponsive pupil □ History of glaucoma/other problems	□ Pilocarpine 0.5% eye drops in affected eye every 15–30 minutes – pupil will constrict □ Rest and sit upright □ Antinausea drugs if needed □ Seek medical advice and evacuate

Acute iritis (acute uveitis)

The casualty may have had previous attacks and may have a disease such as arthritis.

Symptoms and signs	Treatment
□ Sudden onset of pain □ Reddened eye around cornea □ Watering eyes, blurred vision □ Photophobia □ Small, possibly irregular pupil	□ No specific treatment offshore □ Rest, analgesia □ Steroid eye drops may help, but seek medical advice □ Urgent evacuation

Eyelid infections

Symptoms and signs	Treatment
□ Stye: small boil arising from eyelash follicle – may discharge naturally □ Chalazion: infected gland in eyelid, which may develop into an abscess or nodule affecting vision	□ "Hot spooning": wrap warm, damp cloth around small spoon and press to eye; repeat every few hours □ Antibiotic ointment or drops □ Chalazion may need surgery

DENTAL AND MOUTH DISORDERS

Dental problems and mouth ulcers can be debilitating and reduce a crew member to the role of passenger. All crew should have a thorough dental checkup some months prior to departure, particularly for voyages to remote oceans.

The boat should carry a standard dental repair kit that will contain items such as temporary filling material and some basic tools for simple dental procedures. The other aspect of care is control of symptoms, such as pain, swelling, and infection. Do not extract teeth on a boat unless absolutely necessary.

History and examination

- Examination needs to be done in a safe and stable place (such as a bunk) that is well lit (with a head torch, for example).
- Procedures are easier if they are carried out from behind the head.
- Sinusitis may resemble dental pain. Conversely, dental pain is sometimes felt in the face and ears.

Important points in the history

- Site and severity of pain?
- Fever, feeling unwell?
- History of trauma?
- Any foul tasting discharge or smell from mouth or nose?
- Retrieve knocked out teeth/dentures
- Previous dental problems?

Important points in the examination
Look
- Inspect all teeth – note crowns/fillings
- Check gums, tongue (above and below), and lips for inflammation, swelling, and discharge

Feel
- Check each tooth for looseness, tenderness
- Examine lips, tongue, cheeks for tenderness, swelling, ulcers
- Tap the area over the cheek below the eye and the forehead above the eye, checking for sinusitis

Document findings for each tooth

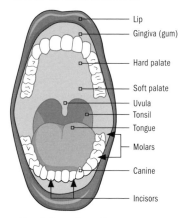

Lip
Gingiva (gum)
Hard palate
Soft palate
Uvula
Tonsil
Tongue
Molars
Canine
Incisors

Front view of mouth

Replacing a filling
- Stable working position; good light; use cotton wool buds to keep tooth/hole dry
- Gently probe cavity, remove loose filling bits
- Push in small amount of filling mix from dental kit (for mixing, follow instructions)
- Pack in firmly and repeat to fill hole (do not leave raised above tooth surface)
- Bite together with damp cotton wool pad between teeth for a few minutes

Specific conditions

Toothache

Symptoms and signs	Treatment
□ May result from cracked tooth or dislodged filling □ Pain on drinking cold/hot drinks □ Pain in tooth or cheek; earache □ May result in root or gum abscess	□ Analgesia □ Antiseptic mouthwash □ Antibiotics in fever and local inflammation □ Replace filling if lost (see p.122)

Root and gum abscesses

Symptoms and signs	Treatment
□ Pain/swelling/inflammation of gum □ May discharge into mouth □ May spread to cause swelling of cheek, difficulty in opening mouth – this is an emergency	□ Oral antibiotics, analgesia □ Antiseptic mouthwash □ Lancing the abscess may be possible if it is tense or pointed □ Seek medical advice if it worsens

Broken or knocked out (avulsed) teeth

Symptoms and signs	Treatment
□ Try to find tooth and keep it in saliva/milk; aim to re-implant within 30 minutes □ Do not handle root of tooth □ Check for other injuries □ Splint broken tooth as for avulsed tooth	□ Clean tooth/socket with sterile saline □ Reimplant to same height as other teeth – hold in place for 10 minutes □ Splint with tin foil wrapped over teeth or filling material squeezed in-between thoroughly dried teeth □ Analgesia and antibiotics

Broken crowns, bridges, and dentures

Symptoms and signs	Treatment
□ There are different types of crowns □ Bridges are also varied and are usually impossible to replace □ Denture wearers should take a spare set; a superglue repair may not be successful	□ It may be possible to reglue a crown – get dental advice □ Clean and dry both surfaces, and use dental glue from the kit □ Sensitive sockets may require temporary filling for protection

Mouth ulcers and cold sores

Symptoms and signs	Treatment
□ May result from trauma (teeth) □ Bacterial infection: bleeding gums and bad breath □ Herpes infection: lots of small ulcers	□ Bacterial infection: antibiotics, antiseptic mouthwash □ Cold sores/herpes virus: oral aciclovir cream early

EAR, NOSE, AND THROAT DISORDERS

Cold, tiring, and damp conditions make boats breeding grounds for infections of the ears, nose, and throat (ENT). Treatment aims to relieve symptoms, while the infection, usually viral, clears in its own time. If there are signs of bacterial infection (pus discharge from nose, ear, or tonsils), give antibiotics.

The various tubes and spaces in the head are good lodging places for foreign bodies, which can cause complications. Diving and air travel to or from the boat may cause pain or rupture of the eardrum (barotrauma) and pain in the sinuses, if they are blocked. A bleeding nose may seem trivial, but can become life-threatening through loss of blood if it is allowed to continue unabated.

History and examination

- Examination needs to be performed in a safe and stable place (such as lying in bunk), with good light (from a head torch, for example).
- Compare sides.
- Do not stick things into the ear, apart from an otoscope. If you do use one, you should make sure you know how to use it the correct way.

Important points in the history

- Site and severity of pain?
- Is pain worse if you: try to exhale with nose blocked/mouth closed; blow nose; tap cheek/forehead?
- Feeling of deafness?
- Feeling of object stuck in throat?
- History of ENT problems?

Outer ear (pinna)

Middle ear
Ear canal   Eardrum   Tube to back of throat (Eustachian tube)

Front view of ear

Important points in the examination

Look (compare sides)
- In ears, up nose, in mouth using good light (otoscope to examine ears if available)
- Pus in ears, on tonsils, in nose
- Inflamed tonsils, throat, ear canal
- Foreign bodies, wax in ears

Feel
- Tap on cheek and forehead – painful with sinusitis

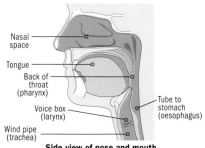

Nasal space

Tongue

Back of throat (pharynx)

Voice box (larynx)

Wind pipe (trachea)

Tube to stomach (oesophagus)

Side view of nose and mouth

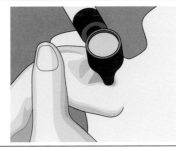
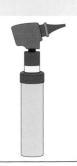

Using an otoscope

- Use an otoscope carefully – stop if you are causing pain
- Gently pull the outer ear upwards and back, to straighten out the canal
- Use a clean tip for each ear and each patient

Specific conditions

Build-up of earwax

Symptoms and signs	Treatment
□ Gradual onset of deafness	□ A few drops of olive oil (or ear drops) each day for a few days □ Do NOT use cotton buds □ May need aspirating by a doctor

Outer ear infection

Symptoms and signs	Treatment
□ Pain and discharge from ear □ Inflamed ear canal, possibly blocked with wax, secretions, swelling □ Pulling on the outer ear hurts □ Feels unwell if severe infection	□ Antibiotic ear drops □ If severe – oral antibiotics □ Gentle cleaning of ear with sterile water □ Avoid diving, swimming, air travel

Middle ear infection

Symptoms and signs	Treatment
□ Pain and deafness □ May feel unwell with cough, cold □ Inflamed eardrum through otoscope □ Eardrum may "pop" – relief of pain, purulent discharge	□ Oral antibiotics □ Painkillers □ Decongestant (pseudoephedrine) may be helpful □ Avoid diving, swimming, air travel

Ear barotrauma

Symptoms and signs	Treatment
□ Pain in ear with changing pressure when Eustachian tube blocked □ Eardrum may be red and inflamed □ Drum may rupture – blood from ear □ If dizzy and sick, seek medical advice	□ Painkillers □ Oral antibiotics if ruptured drum □ Avoid diving, swimming, air travel until better

Foreign bodies in ear, nose, and throat (may need medical help)

Symptoms and signs	Treatment
Ear Deafness, discharge, irritation; an insect may cause buzzing in ear **Nose** Discharge, irritation; danger of inhalation of foreign body **Throat** Coughing, wheezing, may cause choking (*see* pp.44–45); object often stuck at back of tongue, in tonsils; feeling of object in throat may persist	**Ear** Olive oil may soften the object; attempt to remove under direct vision; do not persist and cause injury to canal **Nose** Try to blow out first or remove under direct vision – may need help if far back in nose **Throat** Use tongue depressor and direct vision – use forceps

Sinusitis

Symptoms and signs	Treatment
□ Pain on tapping over cheek below eye, or over forehead above eyebrow □ Fever, headache □ Purulent discharge	□ Oral antibiotics □ Painkillers □ Nasal decongestants

Sore throat and tonsillitis

Symptoms and signs	Treatment
□ Fever, headache □ Some difficulty swallowing □ Tonsillitis – inflamed tonsils, at either side of mouth at back of tongue (use tongue depressor), sometimes with pus visible	□ Use paracetamol, ibuprofen □ Tonsillitis may require antibiotics □ Do not use amoxicillin (or amoxicillin + clavulanic acid) – may cause rash □ If cannot swallow fluids, seek medical advice

Nose bleeds

Symptoms and signs	Treatment
□ Shock may develop with continual bleeding □ Most bleeds are from inside the front part of the nose □ Bleeds from the back of nose are more serious (difficult to control) □ Blood may be swallowed, so not seen on outside □ Check for medications such as warfarin, aspirin, clopidogrel – if the crew is on these, seek medical advice	□ Sit up; do not swallow blood □ Firmly squeeze soft part of nose for 10 minutes; reassess; reapply pressure if needed □ In continued bleeding, cut a ribbon of gauze, soak in paraffin ointment/petroleum jelly; pack firmly into nose, but leave a tail for removal; remove at 48h; seek medical help □ In catastrophic bleeding, pass a lubricated Foley catheter to back of nose, inflate balloon, and pull firmly forwards – only with medical advice

CHEST DISORDERS

Offshore sailing is no longer the preserve of the young and fit. Older crew are more likely to have problems with their heart and lungs, which may be exacerbated by the strains of sailing. Previously unknown problems may come to light in gruelling conditions, even in the young and supposedly fit.

Asthma is a very common example – attacks may be brought on by cold and exercise. Gain an accurate idea of the crew's existing conditions prior to casting off.

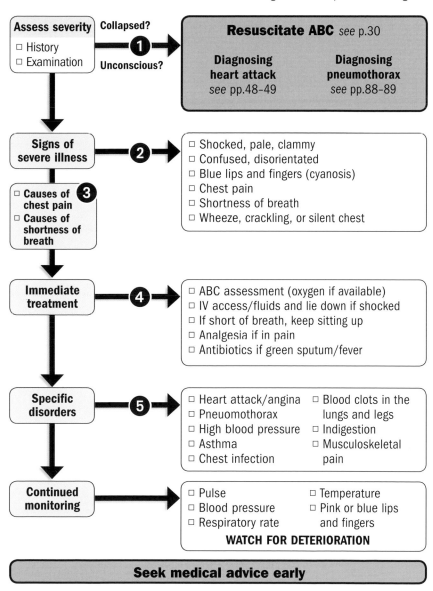

Assess severity
- History
- Examination

Collapsed?

1

Unconscious?

Resuscitate ABC *see p.30*

Diagnosing heart attack *see pp.48–49*

Diagnosing pneumothorax *see pp.88–89*

Signs of severe illness

2

- Shocked, pale, clammy
- Confused, disorientated
- Blue lips and fingers (cyanosis)
- Chest pain
- Shortness of breath
- Wheeze, crackling, or silent chest

- Causes of chest pain
- Causes of shortness of breath

3

Immediate treatment

4

- ABC assessment (oxygen if available)
- IV access/fluids and lie down if shocked
- If short of breath, keep sitting up
- Analgesia if in pain
- Antibiotics if green sputum/fever

Specific disorders

5

- Heart attack/angina
- Pneuomothorax
- High blood pressure
- Asthma
- Chest infection

- Blood clots in the lungs and legs
- Indigestion
- Musculoskeletal pain

Continued monitoring

- Pulse
- Blood pressure
- Respiratory rate

- Temperature
- Pink or blue lips and fingers

WATCH FOR DETERIORATION

Seek medical advice early

❶ History and examination

□ ABC assessment takes priority over everything (see p.30).
□ A blue or very pale patient is a very bad sign – seek medical advice immediately.
□ The casualty may have a history of heart or lung problems.
□ Determine what medications the casualty is taking.

Important points in the history

□ Did the symptoms start suddenly or did they come on over a few days?
□ Pain in the chest:
  - Location (up to jaw, down arms?)
  - Severity (worst ever?)
  - What makes it better or worse?
□ Shortness of breath:
  - Did anything make it worse?
  - Did anything obvious bring it on?
  - Crew able to speak in sentences or just one or two words?
□ Sputum (and colour)
□ Pain/swelling of legs
□ Recent immobility/air travel
□ Any history of similar attacks
□ Normal medications

Important points in the examination

Look
□ Appearance of casualty (blue/white/feverish/sweaty)
□ Obvious struggling with breathing, perhaps sitting upright leaning forwards
□ Tender swelling of calves
Feel
□ Pulse, perfusion
□ Tenderness over chest wall
□ Position of trachea (windpipe)
Listen
□ Breath sounds in the chest using a stethoscope (present or absent?)
□ Harsh or crackly breath sounds
Document
Vital signs, peripheral perfusion

❷ Signs of severe illness

Pale and clammy skin These symptoms are likely to result from severe pain or low blood pressure. There are many causes, including heart attack (see pp.48–49), pneumothorax (see pp.88–89), or severe indigestion (see p.135).

Confusion, disorientation Very low blood pressure, shortage of oxygen, or infections such as meningitis (see p.117) may cause muddled thoughts.

Blue lips or fingers Lack of oxygen or low blood pressure may affect circulation and cause the lips or fingers to turn blue.

Chest pain Pain can be felt anywhere in the chest. If it is crushing, central, and felt in the jaw or down the left arm, it is likely to be coming from the heart.

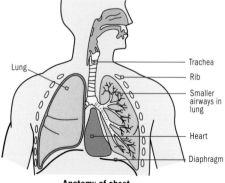

Anatomy of chest

Lung

Trachea
Rib
Smaller airways in lung
Heart
Diaphragm

Shortness of breath Breathing difficulties may manifest as increased rate or deeper breaths. In severe cases, the casualty will be sitting up, bracing themselves forwards with their arms, and the muscles in the neck will stand out with effort.

Wheezing You may not need a stethoscope to hear severe wheezing. It is usually a sign of asthma, but heart problems and chest infections can also cause wheezing.

Crackling Breathing with accompanying crackling sounds can be a sign of chest infection or heart problems.

Silent chest A lack of chest sounds through a stethoscope is very ominous in a casualty who is struggling with their breathing. Seek medical advice immediately.

❸ Causes

Causes of shortness of breath	
□ Asthma	□ Anxiety
□ Pneumothorax	□ Heart problems
□ Pulmonary embolus (blood clot in lungs)	□ Trauma
	□ Chest infection

Causes of chest pain	
□ Heart attack	□ Indigestion
□ Angina	□ Anxiety
□ Pneumothorax	□ Chest infection
□ Pulmonary embolus	□ Trauma

❹ Immediate treatment

If the casualty is having obvious difficulty breathing or has blue lips or fingers, seek medical advice immediately, and start to arrange for immediate evacuation if possible. Use oxygen if available.

Shock Treat shock immediately. Lie the casualty down and prop the legs up above the heart. Insert an IV cannula and give fluids (*see* illustration, right, and pp.172–73) – 500ml initially, then check blood pressure. Seek medical advice immediately.

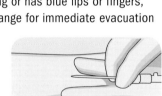
Inserting an IV cannula

Shortness of breath Keep the casualty sitting up – the lungs work better like this. Give oxygen if available. Try to discover the cause of breathlessness – *see* list above and signs/symptoms and treatments of specific conditions.

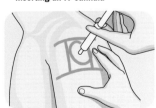
IM injection

Chest pain Pain in the chest should be treated. If very severe, use morphine IM injection (*see* illustration, right, and p.175), otherwise paracetamol and NSAIDs (check no stomach ulcer or asthma problems first).

Try to work out the cause – *see* list above and signs/symptoms and treatments of specific conditions.

Antibiotics Use antibiotics if there is fever and green sputum – intravenously if the casualty looks unwell, has a temperature above 39°C, and is short of breath.

⑤ Specific conditions

Pneumothorax ----------------------------➤ See pp.88–89

Indigestion -------------------------------➤ See p.135

Heart attack/angina

Heart attacks and angina (pain from the heart) are more common with age. Smoking, high blood pressure, diabetes, and previous angina or heart attack all make heart attacks more likely. Angina is less severe than a heart attack, is brought on by heavy work, and should cease when resting. In simple terms, it is the stage before a heart attack and is a sign that the heart is not well. A casualty who suffers from angina should be seen, fully assessed, and treated by a doctor before they board the boat. Voyages to cold climates and isolated oceans may be too hazardous for them.

Symptoms and signs	Treatment
□ Central, crushing chest pain – may also be felt in the left or right arm, jaw, neck, and abdomen □ Pain is continuous with a heart attack □ Pain of angina improves when resting □ Sweating, pale, short of breath □ Nausea and vomiting □ Possible collapse from either low or very high blood pressure	□ **If any doubt, treat as a heart attack** (see pp.48–49) □ Give oxygen if available □ Treat pain with morphine 5–10mg IM injection if very severe, sweaty □ Try glyceryl trinitrate spray (two squirts) under tongue □ If in any doubt, give aspirin 300mg □ Rest and avoid exertion and stress □ Seek medical advice and evacuate

Asthma

Asthma is becoming increasingly common and causes a significant number of deaths – take it seriously. The condition may be precipitated by dust, animals, pollen, cold air, work, infection, and emotion. It may either improve on a boat or worsen, depending on the individual. Prevention and early treatment are key in avoiding problems. Severe asthma and frequent admissions to hospital should preclude long voyages.

Symptoms and signs	Treatment
□ Short of breath, fast respiratory rate □ Wheeze on breathing out □ There may be only slight wheezing in dangerously severe attacks. Look at the casualty – if they look very unwell, they are! □ Barrel chest □ Chest infection and cough □ Pale, exhausted, sitting up, braced □ Unable to talk in sentences (severe if cannot manage a whole sentence) □ Peak flow <50 per cent normal □ **Do not give NSAIDs or betablockers to asthmatics**	□ Keep sitting up and give oxygen □ Give salbutamol inhaler – 4 puffs every 15 minutes □ If not improving, use a spacer or improvise one – inflate a plastic bag, put in 10 puffs of salbutamol, get crew to take 6 breaths □ Continue with salbutamol until crew improves □ Give prednisolone 60mg oral or, in severe attack, put in an IV line and give hydrocortisone 100mg IV □ Give antihistamine (IV or oral) □ Seek medical advice and evacuate

Chest infection (pneumonia)

Chest infections may range from a viral infection, causing irritating cough, to life-threatening pneumonia.

Symptoms and signs	Treatment
□ Fever, feeling unwell □ Short of breath, fast respiratory rate □ Coughing up green sputum □ Possibly wheeze, sharp chest pain □ Crackly, coarse breath sounds	□ If very unwell (respiratory rate >40 breaths per minute, blue colouring), give oxygen if available □ Antibiotics for 5 days (give IV if fever >39°C, very unwell) □ If not improving, seek medical advice

High blood pressure (normal <140/90, severe >160/110)

The casualty may have a history of high blood pressure and will carry medication. Uncontrolled high blood pressure may result from prolonged seasickness (if the casualty has failed to absorb tablets) or from forgetting or losing tablets.

Symptoms and signs	Treatment
□ Headache □ Chest pain □ Nausea, vomiting □ Confusion, fitting if very severe	□ Blood pressure above 160/110 or symptoms – seek medical advice □ Give antinausea drugs and normal medication

Blood clots in the lungs (pulmonary emboli – PE) and legs (deep vein thrombosis – DVT)

Blood clots may form in the leg and thigh veins. These may then float off (embolize) and lodge in the lungs. Large PEs can cause severe chest pain and sudden death. Some crew may be predisposed to blood clots, but they will usually know about it. They may take warfarin and/or aspirin (or may have done so in the past).

The risk increases with obesity, smoking, oral contraceptive pill, pelvic and lower limb fractures, immobility, and dehydration. If the crew collapses with a large PE, there is little you can do except attempt resuscitation.

Symptoms and signs	Treatment
□ Sudden-onset shortness of breath □ Chest pain on one side □ Cough producing bloody sputum □ May be shocked or even in cardiac arrest □ Swollen, tender lower leg or thigh	□ Collapsed – assess ABC (see p.30) □ Give oxygen if available □ Pain relief: IM morphine 5–10mg □ Aspirin 300mg oral □ Seek medical advice and arrange urgent evacuation

Musculoskeletal pain

Pain from a particular point on the chest wall may be quite severe but have no obvious cause, and the crew may be otherwise well. Inflammation of rib/cartilage junctions (costochondritis) may be particularly painful.

Symptoms and signs	Treatment
□ Sudden onset at particular spot □ Pain that may inhibit deep breathing □ Tenderness over the point of pain	□ Exclude other causes □ Analgesia □ Crew may take a few days to improve

ABDOMINAL DISORDERS

Pain and distension of the abdomen while at sea are worrying symptoms, as there are many possible causes; some minor, some more serious. It is crucial to detect signs of infection, abdominal inflammation (peritonitis), and bowel obstruction at an early stage and treat with antibiotics and IV hydration.

Constipation is common on vessels, particularly when freeze-dried food is used; pay continual attention to proper hydration. Other causes of abdominal pain include angina, chest infections, urinary tract infections (*see* p.140), gynaecological disorders (*see* pp.136–37), and diabetic complications (*see* pp.58–59).

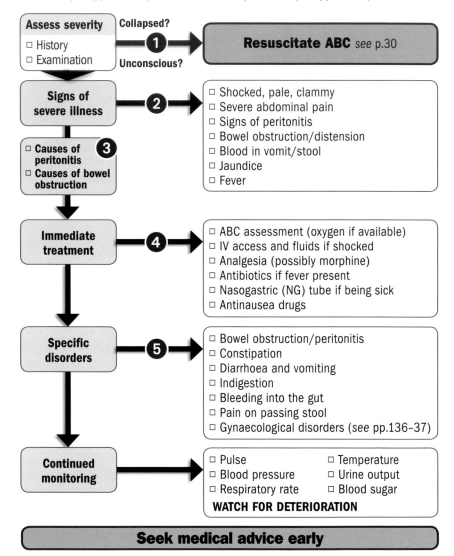

Assess severity
- History
- Examination

Collapsed?

Unconscious?

1 → **Resuscitate ABC** *see* p.30

Signs of severe illness

2 →
- Shocked, pale, clammy
- Severe abdominal pain
- Signs of peritonitis
- Bowel obstruction/distension
- Blood in vomit/stool
- Jaundice
- Fever

3
- Causes of peritonitis
- Causes of bowel obstruction

Immediate treatment

4 →
- ABC assessment (oxygen if available)
- IV access and fluids if shocked
- Analgesia (possibly morphine)
- Antibiotics if fever present
- Nasogastric (NG) tube if being sick
- Antinausea drugs

Specific disorders

5 →
- Bowel obstruction/peritonitis
- Constipation
- Diarrhoea and vomiting
- Indigestion
- Bleeding into the gut
- Pain on passing stool
- Gynaecological disorders (*see* pp.136–37)

Continued monitoring
- Pulse
- Blood pressure
- Respiratory rate
- Temperature
- Urine output
- Blood sugar

WATCH FOR DETERIORATION

Seek medical advice early

❶ History and examination

☐ Symptoms/signs may develop slowly; a casualty may deteriorate over hours or days.
☐ Previous abdominal operations may be significant – look for scars, but remember that the scars of keyhole surgery may be difficult to spot.
☐ Do not carry out a rectal or vaginal examination unless you are trained and have someone to assist you.

Important points in the history

☐ Site and severity of pain?
☐ What makes it better/worse (eating, deep breathing, antacids, vomiting)?
☐ Any nausea/vomiting/diarrhoea/constipation?
☐ Women: menstrual history? Other gynaecological issues? (*see* p.136)
☐ Previous abdominal problems?

Important points in the examination

Look
☐ Feverish, pale, jaundiced?
☐ Abdominal distension?
☐ Scars (look around the umbilicus)?
☐ Blood in vomit or stools?
Feel
☐ Pain with gentle pressing/tapping of the abdomen
☐ Any masses?
Listen
☐ Bowel sounds with stethoscope
Document vital signs, blood sugar, urine output, urine dipstick test

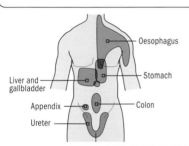
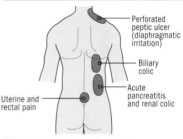

Abdominal pain locations associated with certain organs and disorders

❷ Signs of severe illness

Shocked, pale, and clammy These suggest severe pain or low blood pressure.
Rigid/tender abdomen A rigid, painful, tender abdomen indicates peritonitis.
Bowel obstruction Vomiting of green bile, absence of faeces or flatulence (wind) being passed, and abdominal distension all suggest bowel obstruction.
Blood in vomit/stool Blood in vomit (fresh, or blackish – like coffee grounds) signifies bleeding from stomach or first part of small bowel. Blood in the stool, which may be black and very smelly, may come from piles or the lower bowel.
Jaundice A liver problem is the usual cause of jaundice – often gallstones.
Fever Infection, indicated by fever, may mean that the bowel is very sick and may have perforated or that an infection has affected the kidney.

❸ Causes

Causes of peritonitis

☐ Bowel perforation ☐ Pancreatitis
☐ Appendicitis   ☐ Gallstones
☐ Peptic ulcer   ☐ Gynae. problems

Causes of bowel obstruction

☐ Severe   ☐ Previous surgery
  constipation   ☐ Twisted bowel
☐ Pancreatitis   ☐ Hernia

④ Immediate treatment

Shock Treat shock immediately. Lie the casualty down and prop the legs up above the heart. Insert an IV cannula (*see* pp.172–73) and give IV fluids (500ml initially – measure blood pressure). Seek medical advice immediately.

Analgesia Give the casualty something for the pain. Morphine or tramadol IM may be used to treat severe pain. Do not use NSAIDs until you are certain there is no peptic ulceration or bleeding.

Antibiotics Administer antibiotics at an early stage if there are any signs of infection (temperature over 37.5°C, acute abdomen, bowel obstruction). Give IV if the crew is vomiting or the temperature is over 39°C. Use a broad-spectrum antibiotic and metronidazole (*see* p.206).

Nasogastric (NG) tube The tube should be left open and attached to a bag, to allow the stomach to drain, reducing pain, distension, and vomiting.

Antinausea medication Administer antinausea drugs to reduce vomiting and also when using morphine or tramadol. The medical kit may contain several types; seek medical advice regarding which drugs to use.

⑤ Specific conditions

Bowel obstruction/peritonitis (acute abdomen)
These are life-threatening conditions and need to be detected at an early stage. Treatment can be successful on a boat, containing the cause (which may well not be known) until urgent evacuation can be arranged.

Symptoms and signs	Treatment
□ Severe abdominal pain □ Pain on gentle pressing or tapping □ Rigid abdomen, possibly distended □ Fever □ Vomiting (green bile) □ Check for hernia – painful swelling in groin at top of leg □ "Tinkly" bowel sounds or silence □ Check blood sugar and chest for signs of angina, infection	□ ABC assessment if collapsed □ IV access and 500ml fluid □ Treat severe pain with morphine or tramadol. Seek medical advice □ Antibiotics intravenously □ Antinausea drugs □ Antacid treatment (*see* Indigestion treatment, opposite page) □ NG tube (*see* p.186) and drain bag □ Watch urine output – aim for minimum 0.5ml/kg/hour

Constipation
Freeze-dried food must be properly rehydrated. Normal bowel habit varies enormously, from 3 stools per day to one stool every 3–4 days.

Symptoms and signs	Treatment
□ No stools (or very little hard stool) passed for 2–3 days longer than normal for that crew □ Cramping abdominal discomfort □ Distended abdomen if severe	□ Avoid by good hydration and high-fibre diet (aim for dilute urine) □ Treat with glycerine suppositories, stool softener (lactulose), and stimulants (bisacodyl)

Diarrhoea and vomiting

The cause is usually food poisoning; rarely, an abdominal disorder. Nausea and vomiting alone may indicate seasickness or even pregnancy. Observe strict hygiene.

Symptoms and signs	Treatment
□ Vomiting or diarrhoea or both □ Abdominal cramps □ Dehydration □ Vomit may be yellow, green, bloody □ Stool may be watery, black, or bloody	□ Keep hydrated – rehydration drinks □ IV fluid may be needed if severely dehydrated and still vomiting □ Antinausea drugs (cyclizine) □ Antidiarrhoeal drugs (loperamide)

Indigestion

Indigestion is a frequent occurrence on boats due to a change in diet, irregular and rapidly eaten meals, stress, and fatigue. The pain of severe indigestion may be mistaken for a heart attack (and vice versa).

Symptoms and signs	Treatment
□ Pain over upper part of abdomen or in chest □ Pain may be burning or gripping □ Stomach acid may reflux into mouth	□ Simple antacids □ Medications that reduce acid in stomach (ranitidine, lansoprazole)

Bleeding into the gut

The likely causes of blood in vomit are a bleeding stomach or a duodenal ulcer. Blood in or on stool is most likely to have come from bleeding piles or from another part of the lower bowel. Treatment is limited and the casualty should be evacuated.

Symptoms and signs	Treatment
□ Vomit containing fresh blood or blood like coffee grounds □ Fresh blood on the surface of the stool or tarry black stool (malena) □ Shock may develop □ Inspect around anus if blood on stool or on toilet paper □ History of peptic ulcer disease	□ IV access and 500ml fluid if shocked – seek medical advice □ Medications that reduce acid in stomach (ranitidine, lansoprazole); use type that is absorbed in the mouth □ Monitor urine output – aim for minimum 0.5ml/hour/kg □ Seek medical advice and evacuate

Pain on passing stool

This is very unpleasant, can be excruciating, and may result in avoidance of passing stool and serious constipation. Simple treatments on the boat can be effective.

Symptoms and signs	Treatment
□ Pain on passing stool, worse with hard-formed stool □ Traces of blood on the stool □ Piles may come out of anus □ An anal fissure may be visible	□ Keep hydrated to keep stool soft □ Avoid constipation (see p.134) □ Analgesia – lidocaine gel rubbed up inside the anus before passing stool may help

GYNAECOLOGICAL DISORDERS

There are several concerns that may be caused by the female reproductive organs, as both part of their normal function (menstruation, pregnancy) and as a result of disease (infection).

Examining a fellow crew member in such a sensitive area requires trust and confidentiality on both sides. Internal examination of the vagina is unlikely to be of benefit unless you are trained and have experience. If in doubt about whether to proceed, seek medical advice.

Menstruation and contraception

Normal menstruation (a cycle of four weeks or so) may require some thought before leaving the dock. There are options to control or even suppress the cycle completely, should the woman choose to do so. Consultation with the family doctor six months before a long voyage will allow time for new contraception and cycle control to be tried and changed if necessary. There are several alternatives to the pill for long-term contraception and suppression of menstruation:

Depot injection Injections provide contraception for three months. Spotting may occur during the first three-month treatment, followed by menstruation suppression.

Implant Contraceptive implants provide contraception for up to three years and can be removed at any time. Spotting may occur in the first three months. Menstruation will be suppressed after that.

Intrauterine (IU) contraceptive device IU devices are inserted into the uterus, providing contraception immediately and reducing menstrual bleeding after three to six months.

Pregnancy

Pregnancy causes profound change in a woman's body, and some symptoms may require treatment on the boat. Complications related to pregnancy may occasionally be serious, causing severe abdominal pain and heavy vaginal bleeding. The two disorders of most concern are miscarriage and ectopic pregnancy (*see* p.137). Seasickness may be exacerbated by pregnancy; seek medical advice before giving antinausea medication.

History and examination

☐ Be diplomatic and respect confidentiality.

☐ Gynaecological disorders may be the cause of an acute abdomen and collapse.

☐ Do not perform vaginal examination unless you are trained to do so.

☐ Is there a history of gynaecological problems?

☐ Do a pregnancy test at an early stage, if you have a testing kit on board. These tests are easy to do and provide immediate results.

Female reproductive organs

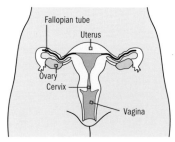

Fallopian tube
Uterus
Ovary
Cervix
Vagina

Important points in the history	Important points in the examination

□ Pelvic or abdominal pain?
□ Possibility of pregnancy?
□ Bleeding or discharge from vagina?
□ Change to menstrual cycle
  – Absent or bleeding mid-cycle?
  – More blood than normal/pain?
□ Pain and frequency passing urine?
□ Method of contraception?
□ Number and outcome of any
  previous pregnancies?
	Look
	□ Pale, in pain, shocked, feverish?
	□ Check discharge (on a pad)
	Feel
	□ Abdomen for tenderness and rigidity,
	  swelling arising out of pelvis
	Listen
	□ Bowel sounds through stethoscope
	Document vital signs, pregnancy test,
	urine dipstick test

Specific conditions

Vaginal bleeding

The normal menstrual cycle may become irregular with stress, fatigue, change of contraception, or pregnancy. Unexpected bleeding may be caused by miscarriage, ectopic pregnancy, intercourse, or infection. Seek medical advice.

Symptoms and signs	Treatment
□ Signs of shock – pale, sweaty, cold □ Tender abdomen □ Try to quantify blood loss – clots? □ Pregnancy test and urine dipstick	□ Treat shock with IV fluids □ Analgesia □ Ergometrine and oxytocin may reduce bleeding in miscarriage

Ectopic pregnancy

This is where the fertilized egg implants in the Fallopian tube, before it arrives at the uterus. As the embryo grows, it causes pain and eventually may rupture the tube, causing serious bleeding into the abdomen but perhaps only a little from the vagina.

Symptoms and signs	Treatment

□ Signs of shock – pale, sweaty, cold
□ Severe abdominal pain (one-sided)
□ Usually happens around week 6–8
  after last period
□ Pregnancy test usually positive
	□ Treat shock – lie down/legs raised
	□ IV fluids – give 1L and seek medical
	  advice
	□ Analgesia
	□ Arrange urgent evacuation

Vaginal discharge

Offensive green, yellow, or watery discharge, vaginal discomfort, and pain on passing urine are all signs of infection. A foul, black discharge may be caused by a forgotten tampon. The discharge should settle once the tampon is removed, but antibiotics may be required if the casualty is feverish and unwell.

Symptoms and signs	Treatment

□ Change in colour/amount of discharge
□ Fever, feeling unwell, frequency of
  urination
□ Abdominal pain or discomfort
	□ If there is white thick discharge, treat
	  for thrush (clotrimazole pessary)
	□ Treat infections with ciprofloxacin
	  and metronidazole

URINARY, KIDNEY, AND GENITAL DISORDERS

Disorders of the male and female genitals are more frequent on boats, where regular washing is more difficult, and may be a serious threat to health.

Infection of the urinary tract is a common problem, more so in women for anatomical reasons. Both male and female genitalia can also become infected and may become extremely uncomfortable and painful. Some of these infections may be sexually transmitted, so it is sensible to practice safe sex and use condoms. Infections affecting the kidney may make the crew very unwell, and possibly shocked, with a high fever. If you suspect a kidney infection, seek medical advice.

The male testes in the scrotum are prone to injury, torsion, and infection, all causing considerable pain. Torsion of the testes is an emergency, requiring surgery within 12 hours if possible. Examination requires trust and confidentiality on both sides. If you have any doubt about what you should examine, seek medical advice.

Passing blood

Blood in the urine can be alarming, particularly when the urine is completely red – an appearance that may be caused by relatively little blood. Reassure the casualty, and treat according to possible cause. The casualty is unlikely to become shocked due to blood loss in the urine. However, if the bleeding continues for a number of days, the casualty may start to become anaemic – displaying symptoms such as paleness, lethargy, and malaise. If this is the case, seek medical advice and arrange evacuation.

Causes of blood in the urine
- Infection of the urinary tract – *see* p.140
- Renal stones – *see* p.141
- Vaginal bleeding colouring the urine
- Trauma (such as pelvic fracture, *see* pp.96–97, or as a result of inserting a urinary catheter), which should settle
- Use of medications such as warfarin, aspirin, clopidogrel, apixaban, etc. – seek medical advice if this is the case
- Other diseases of the kidneys and renal tract – refer to a doctor once on shore
- Red colouration of the urine may be caused by drugs (rifampicin) and foods such as beetroot (in large quantities)

History and examination

- Be diplomatic and respect confidentiality.
- Do not perform a vaginal or rectal examination unless trained to do so.
- If there is genital infection, sexual partners may also be infected. This may cause embarrassment, but the problem must be dealt with. Be as sensitive as possible.

Important points in the history

- Site and severity of pain (including testicles, scrotum, and abdomen)
- Amount and colour of discharge
- Pain and frequency passing urine
- Colour and smell of urine
- Any sores, swellings, or ulcers on genitals or around anus
- Sexual contacts
- Test urine with dipstick
- Pregnancy test for women

Important points in the examination

Look
- Appearance (pale, in pain, feverish, shocked)
- Inflammation, sores, lumps, discharge
- Swollen, reddish-blue scrotum

Feel
- Lower abdomen for tender or swollen bladder
- Flanks for tenderness over kidney
- Scrotum and testicles for swelling and tenderness

Specific conditions

Urinary retention

The most common causes on a boat are infection, pelvic or genitalia trauma, blood clot in the bladder, drugs (antihistamines and some anti-depressants), and loss of consciousness if prolonged. A catheter

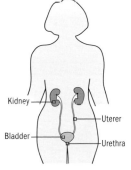

Female urinary tract

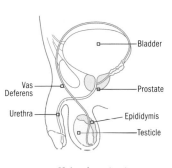

Male urinary tract

must be passed into the bladder through the urethra (see p.187). This should not be attempted if there is blood in the urine following trauma; the alternative is a suprapubic catheter. Inserting a suprapubic catheter is a specialized procedure (see p.188) and you must seek medical advice for guidance.

Symptoms and signs

- Inability to pass urine despite urge to do so
- Fullness and tender lower abdomen
- History of trauma
- Signs of infection

Treatment

- Seek medical advice first before attempting to insert a catheter – it might make matters worse
- A suprapubic catheter may be required (see p.188)
- Leave catheter in and evacuate

Scrotal pain/testicular torsion

The pain of testicular torsion, or twisting, comes on suddenly, is very severe, and may cause the casualty to vomit. The pain is caused by lack of blood supply to the testis. The testis will die unless the twisting is undone quickly (within 12 hours). Usually this is done surgically, which is obviously not possible on a boat. Manual untwisting can be attempted under medical guidance, but may not be successful.

Symptoms and signs	Treatment
□ Sudden-onset, severe testicular pain □ Very tender testis on gentle palpation □ Scrotum may become red and swollen □ No history of trauma – pain may cause the casualty to wake	□ Strong analgesia and antinausea medication □ Seek medical advice and attempt manual untwisting □ Evacuate urgently whether successful or not

Manual untwisting of a torted testis
- □ Position the casualty lying down in a bunk with the scrotum elevated
- □ Gently but firmly hold affected testis in fingers and rotate towards the inner thigh on that side (that is; rotate his right testis anticlockwise, as you look at it, and his left testis clockwise). These are the directions that work most often.
- □ Relief of pain will be immediate, but more than one turn may be necessary
- □ Try rotating in the opposite direction if pain increases

Scrotal pain/epididymitis

Part or all of the testis may become inflamed. The usual cause is infection, possibly sexually transmitted. Only one testis is usually involved. It is important to differentiate from testicular torsion – seek medical advice if any doubt.

Symptoms and signs	Treatment
□ Gradual onset of pain from one testis □ Scrotum may become red and swollen □ Fever, and pain passing urine □ Urine dipstick may show blood and protein in the urine	□ Pain may be relieved by casualty lying down and gently elevating scrotum (e.g. on a rolled-up towel) □ Analgesia □ Antibiotics if signs of infection

Urinary tract infection

Infection may affect all parts of the urinary tract, from the urethra to the kidney. They are common in both sexes, but more so in women. Infections of the kidney may cause the casualty to be very unwell, with a high fever, possible sepsis, and shock.

Symptoms and signs	Treatment
□ Fever □ Kidney infections – very unwell, possibly shocked, flank pain □ Pain and frequency on passing urine □ Urine dipstick – positive for protein, blood, white cells, nitrites	□ If in shock – IV access/fluid and seek medical advice □ Analgesia □ Antibiotics (IV if very unwell) □ Keep hydrated – aim for dilute urine

Kidney (renal) stones
Regularly becoming dehydrated at sea in a hot climate may cause stones to form in the kidney, resulting in severe pain – in the flank and down to the groin – when they are passed. Stones may become lodged in the ureter or bladder, causing obstruction. Infection may cause blood in the urine.

Symptoms and signs	Treatment
□ Sudden severe pain in one flank □ Nausea and vomiting, fever □ Dipstick testing may show blood, protein, nitrites, and white cells	□ Keep well hydrated □ Analgesia – paracetamol, NSAIDs □ Antibiotics if feverish □ Seek medical advice if the symptoms do not improve

Sexually transmitted infections (STIs)
Some STIs are very serious (syphilis, HIV), whereas others are more easily treated (chlamydia, gonorrhoea), but any STI is a serious matter. Sexual contacts must be traced and treated, despite the potential embarrassment. If you have a suspected STI, avoid all sexual contact (including oral contact).

Symptoms and signs	Treatment
□ Green, offensive discharge from penis or vagina □ Pain passing urine, sores on genitals	□ Likely that the cause will not be identified on the boat □ Antibiotics (such as ciprofloxacin)

Genital sores and lumps
Ulcers, blisters, and sores are usually the result of infection, possibly an STI. Herpes blisters and ulcers tend to be numerous and painful. They will usually be preceded by mild tingling, which is when to apply aciclovir cream. Syphilitic ulcers tend to be single, painless, hard-edged, and clean. Bacterial infection may cause swellings and abscesses (possibly in the labia); these may self-discharge but sometimes need antibiotics and even surgical intervention. Genital warts and the small white lumps of molluscum contagiosum do not require treatment on the boat, but avoid sexual contact, and do not share towels or bed linen.

Foreskin problems
The foreskin may become very swollen if it is pulled back over the head of the penis and not put back again. Infection may cause inflammation of the end of the penis under the foreskin, due to an STI or poor personal hygiene.

Symptoms and signs	Treatment
□ Swollen, retracted foreskin – may be very enlarged □ Inflammation and whitish discharge under foreskin. There may be pain on passing urine	□ Lidocaine gel on foreskin for pain, then gentle, long squeeze to reduce swelling. Return foreskin to usual position □ Infection – thorough, regular washing under foreskin. Clotrimazole cream/antibiotics if not improving/severe

INFECTIONS

Once at sea, a boat is an isolated environment and new infections cannot find a way on board. However, what goes on board stays on board, so pay attention to vehicles of infection when in port.

Vehicles of infection

Food and milk Undercooked or untreated food and milk are especially risky.
Water To minimize contamination, make sure all water is clean or treated before it goes into the tanks. It may be advisable to boil drinking water.
Clothing and bedding Micro-organisms and larger pests may inhabit linen.
Crew Members of the crew may be harbouring infections, such as food poisoning, sexually transmitted infections (STIs), and flu.

Prevention

Behaviour Actions are a matter of personal responsibility. Do not get on the boat if you know you have a transmissible disease. Maintain a high level of personal hygiene on the boat and be scrupulously clean when cooking.
Boat cleanliness Hygiene is essential. Establish a rotation in which each crew member shares responsibility for cleaning the entire inside of the boat daily.
Vaccinations Either vaccinations or boosters are recommended before travel to most foreign countries. A certificate of yellow fever immunization is required for entry into some ports. Prophylaxis is required for malaria.
Travel Infections such as malaria and rabies may be endemic in places outside the port. Assess the risks and take adequate precautions.
Anti-bite measures Precautions such as mosquito nets, long trousers, long-sleeved shirts, and insect repellent may be required in some ports, and certainly when travelling to areas where mosquitos are common.
Contamination Contact with bodily fluids, particularly blood, should be avoided. Wear gloves when dealing with wounds.
Wound care In general, inspect and re-dress wounds each day (using clean hands, sterile gloves, and a sterile dressing).

Treatment

Treatment is aimed at controlling the infection and preventing transmission.
Isolation Avoid using the same bedding, towels, and clothes in order to reduce transmission risk. If a particular crew has immunity to a disease, such as chickenpox, they alone should attend to the sick crew.
Hygiene Cleanliness is vital to prevent infection spreading. Skin infections such as impetigo may run riot if hygiene is substandard.
Antibiotics After all precautions have been taken, antibiotics are the final measure. In general, signs of infection should be treated more readily on a boat in the middle of the ocean than on shore, because the consequences of leaving the infection untreated are more serious.

Infections	Organism	Location	Transmission	Symptoms and Signs	Treatment	Vaccine
Malaria	Protozoa	Africa, Americas, Asia, Southern Europe	Mosquito	Incubation 7 days–several months. High fever daily, sweating, headache, muscle aches, diarrhoea, jaundice, shock, fitting, coma, heart failure	If symptoms, seek medical advice and evacuate urgently. Avoid mosquito bites. Consider doxycycline, proguanil, and atovaquone	No, but protective drugs recommended. Seek advice
Yellow Fever	Virus	Africa, South America	Mosquito	Incubation 3–7 days. Headache, fever, chills, aches, vomiting, stomach pain, jaundice, gut bleeding, shock	No direct treatment. Support symptoms, treat shock, and evacuate urgently	Yes, mandatory in some countries
Hepatitis A	Virus	Mostly developing countries	Faecal-oral route (unwashed food)	Fever, chills, vomiting, fatigue, jaundice, pale stool, dark urine	Support symptoms, hydrate, isolate until crew shows improvement, no alcohol	Yes
Typhoid/ Paratyphoid	Bacteria	Widespread (common in Asia)	Faecal-oral route (unwashed food)	Incubation 8–21 days. Fever, headache, cough, abdominal pain, diarrhoea/ constipation, blanching rash on abdomen, gut bleed, shock	Isolate; strict hygiene to prevent spread; antibiotics – ciprofloxacin. Seek medical advice (symptoms similar to malaria) and evacuate	Yes
Dengue Fever	Virus	Southeast Asia, South America, Caribbean	Mosquito	Fever, headache, aches, blotchy rash that blanches, rarely bleeding from nose and gut, shock	Support symptoms, control fever, and hydrate. Evacuate if severe and bleeding. Avoid mosquitos	No
Worm infections	Various worms	Americas, Asia, Africa	Infected water, lakes, rivers; faecal-oral route	Worms seen in faeces and vomit. Skin rashes and anal itching at night. Some worms cause serious illness	Do not bathe in infected water. Strict hygiene. For known infections mebendazole	No
Infestations	Lice, fleas and mites (scabies), and ticks	Widespread	Clothes, bedding, sexual contact, animals (domestic pets and wild)	Itching of head, groin, skin, infected bites; scabies – long burrows between fingers, wrists. Other diseases may be transmitted by fleas, lice, and ticks, including typhus, Lyme disease, plague, tick-borne encephalitis (TBE)	Malathion/maldison orally for scabies and lice. Antihistamine for itch. Thorough treatment with long-acting insecticide in boat for fleas. Gently remove ticks with tweezers. Watch for other symptoms of disease	No (vaccine available for Lyme disease and TBE)

SEASICKNESS: ASSESSMENT

Seasickness among crew is not only debilitating for the individual but may seriously impair the running of the ship and even place it in danger. It is therefore imperative to assess the extent of motion sickness in the ship's crew and institute effective management prior to sailing. In more than 95 per cent of sailors, seasickness can be prevented or treated effectively. The majority will have gained their sea legs within 72 hours.

Once seasickness has become established, frequent reassessment of the situation and appropriate action will, in the vast majority of cases, prevent a drama from becoming a crisis.

Structured assessment

Are you **feeling** sick?	No ❶ ➤	Duties of non-sick crew
Yes ↓		
Are you **being** sick?	No ❷ ➤	Treatment of nausea
Yes ↓ ❸ ↓		
Have you been sick for **>12 hours**?	No ❹ ➤	Initial treatment of vomiting
Yes ↓		
Have you been sick for **>24 hours**?	No ❺ ➤	Ongoing treatment of vomiting
Yes ↓		
Have you been sick for **>72 hours**?	No ❻ ➤	Treatment of severe vomiting
Yes ↓ ❼ ↓		
Treatment of intractable vomiting, which may become life-threatening		

❶ Duties of the non-sick crew

Crew members who are resistant to sickness may have to take on the duties of those who are ill, such as deck work, going below to navigate, and cooking. Sufferers may be uncoordinated and, in severe cases, disorientated. Somebody should be responsible for ensuring that their harnesses are secure at all times, that they do not fall over the side while vomiting, and to supply a bucket, wet wipes, a water bottle, and dry biscuits. Seasick crew may be encouraged to helm, as they can ride with the motion of the ship and watch the horizon, hastening sea legs adaptation.

❷ Treatment of nausea

Crew suffering from nausea should: take oral antiseasickness drugs, get adequate rest and eat small meals frequently; avoid activities such as cooking, navigating, and working on the engine; be positive. For treatment, *see* p.147.

❸ The safe way to be sick

The best place to be sick is in a bucket, which can then be emptied over the side. If being sick over the lee side, clip on and make sure the watch leader knows you are there. Keep an eye on what is happening to the boat and stay safe. Do not, on any account, be sick below, unless into a container, as this will induce vomiting in others.

❹ Initial treatment of vomiting

Continue taking oral antiseasickness medications. It is important to stay hydrated, so continue to take at least fluids by mouth and dry biscuits if possible. Stay warm and dry. If staying on deck, clip on and ask a "buddy" to keep an eye on you. Keep busy if it helps, with activities such as helming.

❺ Ongoing treatment of vomiting (12–24 hours)

Being sick for more than 12 hours will start to be dispiriting, although not for some strange souls! Sufferers will need their spirits supported and should not stay on deck for prolonged periods. Bunks in the middle of the boat are ideal, as motion is minimized. Administer additional types of antiseasickness medications if possible.

❻ Treatment of severe vomiting (24–72 hours)

Oral medications are unlikely to be effective at this point: use tablets that melt and are absorbed in the mouth, or suppositories. Electrolyte replacement fluids should also be used.

❻ Treatment of intractable vomiting (>72 hours)

This situation is serious and may require evacuation. However, with proper treatment, evacuation may be avoided. The risks are: severe dehydration leading to shock; hypothermia; weakness and debilitation; and severe constipation. A thorough assessment of the casualty should be undertaken, including peripheral perfusion (*see* p.167), pulse, blood pressure, and urine output. Injectable forms of antiseasickness medications should be used. Fluid rehydration may be required via IV or rectal routes. **Seek medical advice early**.

SEASICKNESS: PREVENTION AND TREATMENT

"Sit under a tree or in the shadow of an old church" is good advice for the intractable sufferer. For the vast majority, however, seasickness can be effectively controlled.

Cause

The vestibular apparatus (the balance organ in the inner ear), passes movement information to the brain to help it maintain body position and balance. These nerve impulses are reinforced by visual signals and positional sensation from joints. The motion of the boat sends conflicting messages to the brain, which stimulates the seasickness cascade; the exact mechanism is poorly

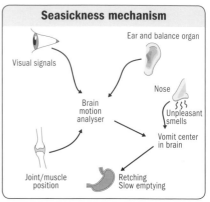

Seasickness mechanism

Visual signals

Ear and balance organ

Nose

Brain motion analyser

Unpleasant smells

Vomit center in brain

Joint/muscle position

Retching
Slow emptying

understood. Extra stimuli, such as smells and tastes, also play a part, as well as cold, anxiety, and fear; but gut symptoms are a secondary phenomenon, so special diets have little effect in preventing the condition.

Symptoms and signs of seasickness

Stomach	Brain
□ Loss of appetite	□ Pallor and sweating
□ Fullness of stomach	□ Dizziness, drowsiness
□ Nausea	□ Yawning, excessive breathing
□ Vomiting/retching	□ Headache, malaise
□ Occasional blood in vomit	□ Dry mouth or increase in saliva

Prevention

□ Avoid heavy meals, alcohol, and recreational drugs before sailing.
□ **Start antiseasickness remedies 12–24 hours before embarking**; suitable drugs should be established before an extended voyage.
□ Sleep on board the night before departure and get a good night's rest.
□ Dress appropriately: wear more clothing than you need rather than less.
□ Keep occupied and do not do chart work, navigate, go below, or cook.
□ Stay in the fresh air. Fix your gaze on land, clouds, stars, or the horizon, which provide a stable reference point. Helm if possible.
□ Keep hydrated, taking small amounts of water (or sugary drink) and small frequent snacks, even if continuing to be sick. There will be some benefit.
□ Finally, be positive and believe in a rapid recovery.

Treatment

There are many medications that aim to control seasickness. They work on a variety of chemical pathways in the brain and gut, and each produces a slightly different effect. Each individual will find a particular medication (or combination of medications) that works, with minimal side effects.

The most commonly used medications are included in the table below. Start at the top of the table, until you find one that is acceptable to you. Do not combine medications that have the same action. If you take prescription medication, it is very important to consult the family doctor before taking any antiseasickness drugs, as they might interact and be harmful.

Medication	Route	Dose	Way it works	Notes
Cinnarizine	Oral	30mg 6-12 hours before departure then 15mg every 8 hours	Antihistamine	Although an antihistamine, usually has little sedative effect
Domperidone	Oral	10-20mg every 6 h	Peripheral antidopamine	Well tolerated, nonsedating. Convert from suppositories once vomiting stops
	Suppository	30mg every 6 h (orally when able)		
Prochlorperazine	Oral	10mg every 6 h	Central antidopamine	Some sedative properties, dry mouth, rarely causes abnormal movements, tremor, and restlessness
	Under tongue	3mg every 6 h		
	IM injection	12.5mg injection, then oral therapy 6 h later		
Hyoscine hydrobromide	Patch behind ear	Replace patch every 72 h, on the opposite side	Anticholinergic	Sedative effects, dry mouth; rarely, difficulty passing urine. Take care with patch as contamination will dilate pupil and blur vision. Wash hands after use.
	Oral	0.3mg every 8 h		
Ondansetron	Oral	4-8mg every 8 h	Antiserotonin	Nonsedating, occasional constiptation
	Under tongue	4-8mg every 8 h		
Cyclizine	Oral	50mg every 8 h	Antihistamine	Slight sedation only. Painful injection
	IM injection	50mg every 8 h		
Promethazine	Oral	25mg every 6-8 h	Antihistamine	Significant sedation, which may be an advantage. Dry mouth; rarely, difficulty passing urine

Alternative treatments

Several alternative treatments may work well for some crew: wrist bands can provide acupressure or electrical pulses over the neiguan (P6) acupuncture point. Ginger root (1g every 8 hours) may also be effective.

SKIN DISORDERS

Sun, saltwater, heat, cold, damp, and manual work all damage the skin. In bad conditions, skin tends to get thicker and less sensitive, particularly on the fingers, which after a week or so may end up looking enlarged (known as "sausage fingers").

It is wise to take simple measures to protect the skin as much as possible before more expensive, complicated treatments become necessary.

Protection measures

Reduce time of sun exposure Always keep in mind how long you have been in the sun.

Protective clothing when exposed Wear a wide-brimmed hat, long sleeves, long trousers, and gloves to protect back of hands when helming/trimming.

Routine sunscreen Use physical screens such as zinc or titanium oxide-based creams or high factor chemical screens (>SPF 15) containing para-aminobenzoic acid or cinnamates. Water-resistant agents are ideal.

Sunglasses Make sure sunglasses have side protection. Goggles or even a helmet with a visor may be needed when very rough.

Gloves When helming, trimming, or doing deck work, wear gloves. Large mitts are particularly good when helming, for warmth.

Shoes or boots Wear foot protection at all times on deck and on shore.

Regular moisturizer Apply moisturizer to hands at the end of each watch. This should not be seen as a "soft" thing to do, but as a means of keeping the hands and fingers in good shape so they function better.

Boat hygiene Cleanliness is essential in reducing infections (*see* p.142).

Personal hygiene Take responsibility for maintaining your own hygiene. Pay particular attention to the feet and groin, which are areas prone to fungal infections. Dry as thoroughly as possible and keep all parts aired.

Clothing Make sure your clothes are free of any infestations (fleas etc.) before getting on the boat. Change as often as practical.

Infections Keep an eye on your own skin and that of others. Intervene early if there are signs of inflammation, rash, itching, spots, boils, or bites.

Specific conditions

Sunburn

Wind, UV light reflected from the surface of the sea, and lack of natural shade all increase the risk of severe sunburn, which is easy to prevent but less easy to treat.

Symptoms and signs	Treatment
□ Red, painful skin on exposed parts	□ Keep hydrated and in the shade
□ Dehydration, malaise, nausea	□ Paracetamol and NSAIDs
□ Crew feels chilly but is hot to touch	□ Hydrocortisone 1% cream may help
□ Blisters and swelling if severe	□ Do not burst blisters

Rashes (including heat rash)

Infection, allergic reactions, and abrasive conditions on board are common causes of rashes of varying types. A nonblanching rash may indicate meningitis – see p.117.

Symptoms and signs	Treatment
□ Red, raised, blotchy, itchy lumps (hives) – likely to be allergic reaction □ Rashes with sores that exude pus are likely to be infective □ Rash in armpits and on waist, chest, and back may be prickly heat	□ Look for source of allergy and treat accordingly (see pp.50–51) □ Infection may be bacterial, viral, or fungal (see below) □ Heat rash – keep area dry and clean. Calamine lotion or hydrocortisone

Skin infections

Impetigo in particular can infect an entire vessel's crew very quickly.

Symptoms and signs	Treatment
Viral (shingles/herpes) – very painful blisters that erupt and crust, usually in one area. Crew unwell prior to rash. **Bacterial** □ Impetigo – crusting blisters that spread in patches; itchy, red, painful □ Cellulitis – painful, red, superficial spreading from a wound site □ Fungal – generally in groin or between toes. Reddish, cracking skin, spreading outwards	**Shingles** Analgesia, antibiotics only if blisters become infected **Impetigo** Strict hygiene (no sharing towels etc). Antibiotics: flucloxacillin and fusidic acid. Seek medical advice if not improving after 3 days **Cellulitis** Antibiotics: amoxicillin + clavulanic acid. Seek medical advice if not improving after 3 days. **Fungal infection** Miconazole cream for 10 days. Keep clean and dry

Salt-water boils, "gunwhale bum," tropical ulcers

Tropical ulcers start from a trivial scratch or wound on the shin, over which a pustule forms, which then discharges after some days, forming a painful, hard-edged ulcer.

Symptoms and signs	Treatment
□ Saltwater boil – a collection of smaller boils join together; usually on arms, hands □ Gunwhale bum – a red, painful rash on the buttocks brought on by damp, warm heat and sitting on the rail □ Tropical ulcers – nonhealing ulcer	□ Saltwater boil – if large/not draining, may need lancing. Antibiotics: amoxicillin + clavulanic acid □ Gunwhale bum – keep dry and aired: analgesia, barrier cream □ Tropical ulcers – antibiotics: amoxicillin + clavulanic acid/metronidazole

Itchy skin

Itching may be caused by an ongoing condition, such as eczema, or by contact with new substances.

Symptoms and signs	Treatment
□ Known condition, known allergy □ New exposure (saltwater, sun, oil, fuel)	□ Remove substance if known □ Antihistamine (loratadine, cetirizine), aqueous creams, emollients

BITES AND STINGS

The source of a bite or sting is often unknown. Most injuries will cause a little pain, itching, localized swelling, and some ongoing discomfort. However, stings sometimes cause an intense allergic response known as anaphylaxis, particularly when a toxin is involved. This condition is life-threatening, with a grave outlook if treatment is not commenced promptly (see pp.50–51).

Animals	Regions where most prevalent
Animals that sting	
☐ Bees, wasps, hornets	All areas
☐ Mosquitoes	Tropical and subtropical
☐ Jellyfish	All areas (except Arctic and Antarctic)
☐ Sea anemones	All areas (except Arctic and Antarctic)
☐ Fire coral	Tropical and subtropical
☐ Portuguese man-of-war	All areas (except Arctic and Antarctic)
Animals that jab with spines	
☐ Catfish	Marine, estuarine, freshwater
☐ Cone shells	Tropical and subtropical
☐ Sea urchins	Tropical and subtropical
☐ Stinging fish (lionfish, scorpionfish, stonefish, needlefish, weeverfish)	Tropical and subtropical (weeverfish – temperate)
☐ Stingrays	Atlantic, Pacific, Indian Oceans Freshwater (South America)
Animals that bite	
☐ Sharks	All areas (except Arctic and Antarctic)
☐ Moray eels	Tropical
☐ Barracuda	Tropical and subtropical
☐ Sea snakes	Tropical and subtropical (fresh and sea)
☐ Crocodiles, alligators	Tropical and subtropical
Particularly dangerous small marine animals that have caused fatalities	
☐ Box jellyfish (sea wasp)	Southeast Asia/northern Australia
☐ Needlefish	Caribbean, western Africa, Japan, Indian Ocean
☐ Irukandji jellyfish	Southeast Asia/northern Australia
☐ Blue-ringed and -spotted octopuses	Indian/Pacific tropics
☐ Flower sea urchin	Indian/Pacific tropics

Prevention

☐ Insect repellent
☐ Splash or shuffle feet in shallow water
☐ Do not wear bright objects in the water
☐ Take care diving at night with a torch
☐ Do not swim if you have open wounds

☐ Do not touch unknown animals or corals
☐ Wear shoes at all times and dive suits
☐ Do not harass animals at anytime
☐ Make sure tetanus vaccination is in-date
☐ Carry antivenom in high risk areas

General symptoms of bites and stings

Typical Symptoms	
□ Pain	□ Rash
□ Stinging	□ Redness
□ Itching	□ Swelling

Unusual Symptoms	
□ Headache	□ Nausea and vomiting
□ Weakness	□ Muscle pain
□ Sweating	□ Chest pain

Anaphylaxis (see pp.50–51)

Symptoms and signs
□ General skin flushing
□ Swelling of lips and eyes
□ Fast pulse
□ Faintness
□ Wheezy chest
□ Shock

Treatment
□ ABC assessment if collapsed
□ Adrenaline 0.5mg IM (0.5ml of 1:1000 solution). Adult dose
□ Antihistamine: chlorphenamine 10–20mg IM
□ Steroid: hydrocortisone 100mg IM/IV
□ IV access/fluids (500ml immediately)

Immediate treatment of bites and stings

If collapsed, difficulty breathing See pp.50–51

If large bite, retrieve casualty from water and treat as trauma See pp.32–33

Stings
- □ Avoid the stings or tentacles – use gloves.
- □ The sting area can be covered with vinegar or bicarbonate, but this may make envenomation and pain worse.
- □ Cover the area with shaving cream, flour, or sand/seawater paste, and scrape a knife across to remove stingers – this avoids any further envenomation.
- □ Soak the area in very warm seawater (as warm as tolerated) for 60–90 minutes. This will encourage the breakdown of venom in the skin.
- □ Thoroughly wash the area, and put sterile dressings on wounds.
- □ For relief of pain – ibuprofen gel and lidocaine 2% gel are effective.
- □ For itching – oral antihistamine (loratadine or cetirizine).
- □ For inflammation – hydrocortisone 1% cream is effective.
- □ Observe the crew and wounds for signs of infection or deterioration.
- □ If signs of infection, apply mupirocin 2% cream 2–3 times a day

Bites and penetrating wounds
- □ Wash the wound thoroughly with soap and hot water (sterile if possible).
- □ Remove embedded spines if possible. DO NOT remove large spines (such as those from a stingray) from the chest, head, neck, or abdomen – bleeding may worsen.
- □ Stop bleeding with direct pressure (see p.70). Avoid using tourniquet if possible.
- □ Soak wound in very warm water (as warm as tolerated) for 60–90 minutes.
- □ Cover wound with sterile dressing and check daily for infection.
- □ Start broad-spectrum antibiotics (amoxicillin + clavulanic acid or ciprofloxacin).
- □ **Check tetanus status and availability of an antivenom.**

OVERDOSES AND POISONING

Prescription drugs and recreational substances can both cause deliberate or accidental overdose.

Carbon monoxide is a risk on any boats with gas stoves or heating, diesel drip heaters, and long hours of engine use, particularly if there is inadequate ventilation or poorly serviced equipment. Chlorine is another potential poison, which may be released if the battery bank floods. Enclosed spaces are always a risk.

It is vital to find out what has been taken and how much, so that severity, treatment, and possible complications can be accurately assessed. Look around and gather evidence such as pill bottles, containers, and prescriptions.

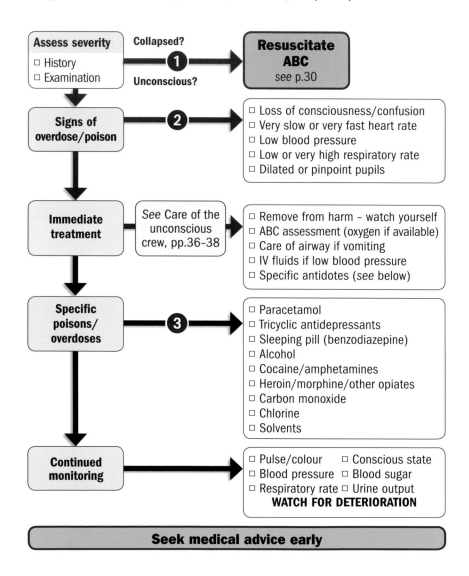

Assess severity
- □ History
- □ Examination

Collapsed?
①
Unconscious?

Resuscitate ABC
see p.30

Signs of overdose/poison
②
- □ Loss of consciousness/confusion
- □ Very slow or very fast heart rate
- □ Low blood pressure
- □ Low or very high respiratory rate
- □ Dilated or pinpoint pupils

Immediate treatment
See Care of the unconscious crew, pp.36–38
- □ Remove from harm – watch yourself
- □ ABC assessment (oxygen if available)
- □ Care of airway if vomiting
- □ IV fluids if low blood pressure
- □ Specific antidotes (see below)

Specific poisons/ overdoses
③
- □ Paracetamol
- □ Tricyclic antidepressants
- □ Sleeping pill (benzodiazepine)
- □ Alcohol
- □ Cocaine/amphetamines
- □ Heroin/morphine/other opiates
- □ Carbon monoxide
- □ Chlorine
- □ Solvents

Continued monitoring
- □ Pulse/colour   □ Conscious state
- □ Blood pressure □ Blood sugar
- □ Respiratory rate □ Urine output
  WATCH FOR DETERIORATION

Seek medical advice early

➊ History and examination

☐ Make sure you do not become poisoned yourself.
☐ If everyone is ill, consider carbon monoxide/chlorine fumes in the cabin.
☐ Look around for empty pill bottles/packets/prescriptions/syringes/needles.

Important points in the history	Important points in the examination
☐ The casualty may be able to tell you everything ☐ Ask about previous medical problems ☐ Normal medications – check whether any are "slow-release" forms. The casualty may get worse ☐ Alcohol is often taken with a deliberate overdose	**Look** ☐ Conscious state (confusion) ☐ Very pink or pale ☐ Pupils – large or small/reactive **Feel** ☐ Peripheral perfusion ☐ Brisk reflexes, tremor **Document** blood sugar, consciousness

➋ Signs of overdose

Opiates (morphine/heroin): Loss of consciousness (LoC), low blood pressure (BP), low respiratory rate, very small pupils
Tricyclic antidepressants: LoC, fast heart rate (hr), large pupils, brisk reflexes
Sleeping pills (benzodiazepine), alcohol, tricyclic antidepressants (severe): LoC, low BP, low respiratory rate, smallish pupils, floppy
Cocaine, amphetamines: Agitation, tremor, sweating, fast hr, nausea, fever, big pupils
Carbon monoxide poisoning: LoC, low BP, fast respiratory rate, stiff muscles, brisk reflexes, pale or flushed (cherry red)

➌ Specific conditions

In all cases, if symptomatic, seek medical advice and evacuate urgently.
Paracetamol
Paracetamol is dangerous in overdose. It has no initial effect (the casualty appears normal), but poisons the liver over several days. Seek medical advice.

Tricyclic antidepressants
These drugs come in many different forms but have similar effects in overdose.

Symptoms and signs	Treatment
☐ LoC, confusion, large pupils, fever ☐ Fast hr but low BP with large overdose	☐ Supportive – keep airway clear and ensure vomit is not inhaled. ☐ May need IV fluid if low BP

Sleeping pills (benzodiazepines – temazepam, diazepam, nitrazepam)
Benzodiazepines in overdose will anaesthetize the casualty.

Symptoms and signs	Treatment
☐ Sleepy, then LoC ☐ Low BP and respiratory rate ☐ Smallish pupils, relaxed muscle tone	☐ Supportive – keep airway clear and ensure vomit isn't inhaled ☐ Flumazenil is an antidote, but seek medical advice first

Alcohol
Overdose of alcohol (usually spirits) is common. Pills are often taken at the same time.

Symptoms and signs	Treatment
□ Sleepy then LoC, smallish pupils □ Low BP, respiratory rate, blood sugar □ Look for other poisoning signs	□ Supportive – keep airway clear □ May need IV fluid if BP is low □ May need sugar (not oral in LoC)

Cocaine/amphetamines
Major overdoses of cocaine and amphetamines may result in LoC, which is grave.

Symptoms and signs	Treatment
□ Agitation, tremor, sweating, heat □ Fast hr, dilated pupils □ Fitting, in severe overdose	□ Keep cool – tepid cloths, fan □ IV access and fluids □ Seek medical advice

Opiates (morphine, heroin)
Opiates may be taken by mouth, smoked, or injected.

Symptoms and signs	Treatment
□ Pinpoint pupils, sleepy, then LoC □ Low BP and respiratory rate □ Look for injection marks, needles	□ Supportive – keep airway clear □ Naloxone is an antidote, but should be given under medical supervision

Carbon monoxide poisoning
Poisoning by carbon monoxide has an insidious onset – entire crew may be affected.

Symptoms and signs	Treatment
□ Lethargy, headache, nausea, vomiting □ Fast respiratory rate, chest pain □ Low BP and LoC, possible fitting □ Pale or (more serious) flushed □ Outlook is grave in LoC	□ Watch yourself □ Get casualty on deck, give oxygen □ Supportive – clear airway □ Treat fitting (see p.40)

Chlorine
Leaking battery acid can cause chlorine poisoning – sealed batteries are safer.

Symptoms and signs	Treatment
□ Wheeze, cough, breathless □ Chest pain □ Watering, sore eyes □ Breathlessness may worsen over several hours	□ Watch yourself □ Get casualty on deck, give oxygen □ Salbutamol inhaler 2 puffs/15 mins □ Prednisolone 60mg orally □ Evacuate before casualty worsens

Solvents (methanol, ethylene glycol)
Solvents may cause deliberate or accidental overdose. Label containers clearly.

Symptoms and signs	Treatment
□ Nausea, vomiting, low BP □ Confusion, possible fitting, then LoC □ Low or high blood sugars □ Effects may be delayed up to 36 hours	□ Supportive – keep airway clear □ Check blood sugar (see p.59) □ If methanol or ethylene glycol poisoning, give 150ml gin/vodka/whisky (only if conscious)

PSYCHOLOGICAL DISORDERS

Boats usually bring out the best in crew members, but very occasionally may bring out the worst. It is well advised, particularly when embarking on a long expedition, to gather the crew together beforehand to identify any potential conflict and take note of any crew member who may require help and advice.

Prevention

Being at sea can be physically and emotionally stressful, which may exacerbate tensions. If disagreements or conflicts cannot be resolved prior to departure, one option is to change crew member, but this is a last resort. It is essential to know about any problems that crew member may have been treated for in the past, such as depression or anxiety attacks.

Prevention strategies include:

□ Recognizing tiredness, getting enough sleep, cating and drinking properly
□ Understanding that everything does not always run smoothly and that plans change
□ Making sure no crew member becomes isolated or withdrawn
□ Assigning appropriate roles to suit each crew member's capabilities
□ Keeping a sense of humour and a sense of proportion.

Depression

Signs include isolation, withdrawal, poor appetite, poor sleep, lethargy, and tearfulness. The crew member may have been treated for similar episodes in the past. If the crew member normally takes medication for depression, check that he or she is taking the prescribed dose. Ensure the crew member is not isolated and has a friend in whom he or she can confide. Find out if there is a particular reason for the symptoms.

Anxiety and panic attacks

Extreme weather, accidents, the unknown, and the unexpected may lead to anxiety in all but the unaware. Acute anxiety is an exaggerated response of feelings of dread and doom, tearfulness, lack of control, together with physical symptoms of fast heart rate, breathlessness, and dizziness. Once this is recognized as acute anxiety, put the crew member in a safe place (a quiet bunk if there is one) until the crisis is over, and then talk things over with them. Diazepam (5mg orally as needed) may control the symptoms until the emergency passes.

Sleep disorders

Long flights to the boat, changes of time zones, hard work, and disturbed sleep may all combine to cause fatigue, which quickly saps morale and decreases performance. It is important to avoid the downwards spiral of progressively poor sleep, so try to start the voyage well rested. Once underway, the watch system should be imposed as soon as possible, so crew members get regular sleep from the start. After a few days, the body adjusts to shorter, more frequent periods of sleep (such as 3 hours 3 times in 24 hours), but a longer period of sleep (up to 6 hours) is occasionally required.

Emergency Medical Procedures

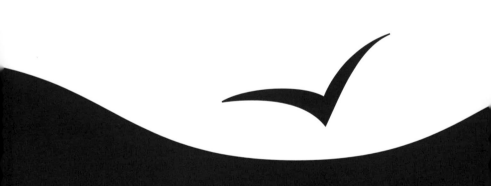

- Resuscitation Procedures
- Recovery Position and Log Roll
- Spinal Immobilization
- Pulse and Blood Pressure
- Assessing Conscious State: Glasgow Coma Scale (GCS) and AVPU
- Rehydration
- Venous and Intraosseus Access
- Injections and Infusions
- Minor Operative Set-up
- Repairing the Skin
- Chest Drains and Emergency Chest Decompression
- Incision and Drainage of an Abscess
- Local Anaesthesia: Nerve Blocks and Infiltration
- Insertion of Tubes and Catheters
- Splints, Casts, and Slings
- Reducing Fractures and Dislocations

RESUSCITATION PROCEDURES

The skills involved in resuscitating a casualty are relatively easy to learn but can make a real contribution towards survival.

Ensure that you have proper training, and practice frequently, so that you will be prepared when you face an unconscious casualty.

Control and stabilization of the cervical spine (neck)

- □ In trauma situations, there may be injury to the cervical spine that is not obvious.
- □ Avoid any unnecessary movement of the head and cervical spine and immobilize (as outlined below) as soon as possible. Sometimes movement is unavoidable, for example if you are removing the casualty from a hazardous position, but try to keep it to a minimum.
- □ Immobilizing the cervical spine manually is only the first step. Full immobilization involves fitting a semi-rigid collar around the neck and strapping the patient to a spinal board (*see* pp.164–65).

Immobilizing the cervical spine with your hands

- □ Manoeuvre firmly but gently. If the casualty is conscious, explain what you are doing.
- □ Do not let go. You are responsible for the position of the cervical spine.
- □ Do not cover the ears with your hands. This is likely to make the casualty feel claustrophobic.

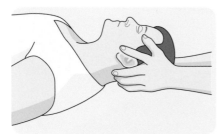

Hold the head without covering the ears, to avoid causing feelings of claustrophobia.

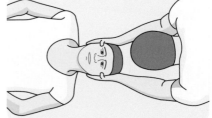

Position yourself comfortably and keep the head as still as possible.

Opening the airway and checking for breathing

There are two basic manoeuvres you can try. Start with the combined head tilt and chin lift. Assess whether you have been successful at opening the airway and whether or not the casualty is breathing:

- □ **Look** at the chest for movement.
- □ **Listen** with your ear next to the mouth for breath sounds.
- □ **Feel** with your cheek next to the mouth for movement of air.

If there are no signs of breathing, try the jaw thrust (*see* opposite page), and reassess the breathing.

Head tilt and chin lift

- Place two fingers under the chin and pull the chin up.
- Put your hand on the forehead and push backwards so the head is tilted as in the diagram.
- If you can, perform these manoeuvres with a pillow or similar padding under the head.

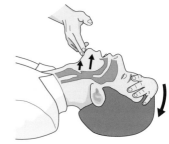

Head tilt and chin lift

Jaw thrust

- Put two fingers behind the "corner" of the jaw, under the ear, on each side.
- Push the jaw forwards, so the lower teeth sit in front of the upper teeth.
- Reassess for breathing.

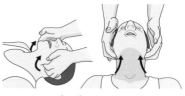

Jaw thrust

Using equipment to keep the airway open

There are two simple devices that are easy to insert and that will help to keep the airway open: oropharyngeal and nasopharyngeal airways. When the casualty is breathing without your assistance, your hands will be free for other things.

Inserting a oropharyngeal airway

- Do not push the tongue back in the mouth.
- Do not insert in a semi-conscious casualty – they may vomit.

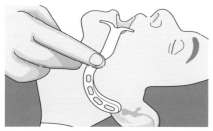

Size the airway – length should match the distance from corner of mouth to ear lobe.

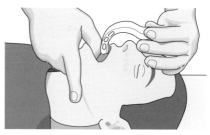

Insert the airway upside down. Do not force.

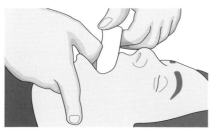

Gradually rotate the device into the correct position up as you insert it.

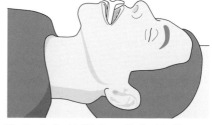

The flange should sit between the front teeth once the airway is in place.

Inserting a nasopharyngeal (NP) airway

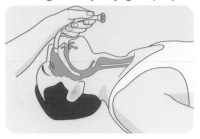

Direct the tube backwards and down.

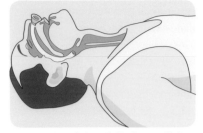

When the airway is in, only the flange will show.

☐ The length of the NP airway should be the same as the distance from the side of the nose to the ear lobe.

☐ Apply lubricant to the airway.

☐ Insert the airway towards the back of the head, not up towards the brain.

☐ When the airway is in place, the flange on the end should lie against the nostril.

☐ If there is a safety pin provided, insert it into the flange before you put the airway in, to prevent the airway from disappearing up the nose.

Note Never use an NP airway if you a suspect a basal skull fracture. Signs of basal skull fracture include: obvious injury to the face; bruising around the eyes; bruising behind the ears; and clear fluid coming from the nose.

How to give rescue breaths

☐ Establish an airway and check for breathing, as outlined in the previous pages.

☐ When performing mouth-to-mouth, use a pocket mask if you can (illustrated below left), to prevent infection. If available, give oxygen through a tube placed under the side of the mask.

☐ You can give rescue breaths positioned at either side of the casualty or above the head. Preserve the airway by maintaining head tilt, chin lift, or jaw thrust.

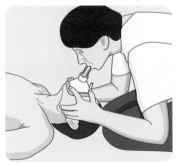

If your medical kit includes a pocket mask, using this will help to prevent infections.

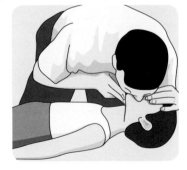

Ensure that the airway remains open, maintaing a head tilt and chin lift if necessary.

☐ Blow into the mask or mouth firmly but gently for 1–2 seconds and watch for the chest rising. Hold the nose at the same time, to prevent the air from escaping.

☐ Aim for the chest to rise an inch or so, then stop blowing and watch it fall.

☐ If you have to blow very hard, and the chest does not rise and fall easily, the airway is not open. Adjust the head position to open the airway.

How to give chest compressions

☐ Lie the casualty facing upwards on a firm surface, taking care of the cervical spine if appropriate.

☐ Assess breathing and pulse (*see* pp.166–67).

☐ Clasp your hands as shown, with the heel of the lower hand on the centre of the chest between the nipples.

☐ With straight arms, push down on the chest, aiming to depress the centre of the chest by two inches (less for smaller adults). Do this at a rate of 100–120 times per minute.

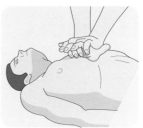

Apply pressure with the heel of one hand.

☐ After 30 compressions, give 2 rescue breaths. Continue with a ratio of 30 compressions to 2 rescue breaths.

Safe defibrillation

☐ Lie the casualty facing upwards on a firm surface, taking care of the cervical spine if appropriate.

☐ Assess the patient for breathing and pulse (*see* pp.166–67). Continue chest compressions until the AED is attached.

☐ Make sure the patient is dry, the surface the patient lies on is dry, and you are dry. Seawater is a very good conductor of electricity.

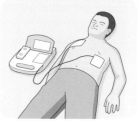

Automated external defibrillator

☐ Attach the defibrillator pads as shown, one just below the collar bone on the right side of the chest and the other below and to the side of the left nipple (not on the breast in women).

☐ Remove the oxygen mask and place it somewhere out of the way.

☐ Turn on the AED and refer to the product manual.

☐ **MAKE SURE EVERYONE IS WELL AWAY FROM THE CASUALTY BEFORE DEFIBRILLATING – THERE IS RISK OF ACCIDENTAL SHOCK**

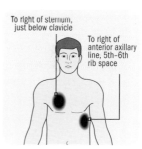

To right of sternum, just below clavicle

To right of anterior axillary line, 5th–6th rib space

☐ After defibrillation, continue with life support – follow the AED instructions.

☐ The AED may give a verbal or "bleep" guide to both the correct rate of compressions and the correct depth of compressions.

Sites for defibrillator pads

RECOVERY POSITION AND LOG ROLL

Recovery position

After an accident or illness, an unconscious or semi-conscious casualty may not be able to maintain their own airway properly. This means that:

- The tongue may fall back and block the airway.
- Saliva may trickle down into the trachea (wind pipe) and lungs.
- Refluxing stomach acid and vomit may also pass into the lungs.

Contamination of the lungs with secretions or vomit will cause a chest infection and threaten recovery. Particularly in an unconscious casualty, stomach acid can reflux into the mouth and then into the lungs without any external sign.

Method

- Ensure the casualty is stable, has an open airway, is breathing, and has a pulse.
- Leave any airway devices in place (see pp.159–60).
- Use the log roll (see opposite page) if there is any suspicion of spinal injury.
- Straighten the casualty's arms and legs, taking appropriate care of the spine. Move the arm closest to you up, so the hand is alongside the head (**1**).
- Bring the opposite arm over, and place the back of the hand against the cheek on your side.
- Bend the opposite leg up at the knee (**2**). With one hand on the bent knee, use the leg as a lever, to gently rotate the casualty towards you. With your other hand, bring the shoulder over at the same time (**3**). Control the rotation with your knees.
- Position the head comfortably on the back of one hand, and bring the bent upper leg over far enough to prevent the body from rolling in either direction (**4**).
- The arms and upper leg should form right angles, for best support.

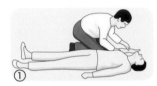
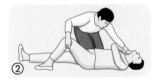
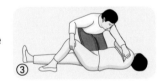
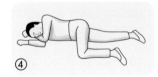

Notes

- Assess for ABC frequently (see p.30) and immediately after turning.
- The recovery position is quite stable, and the casualty can stay in this position for a few hours. If the boat is rolling, place rolled-up sleeping bags or something similar on either side of the casualty.
- Injured limbs may need extra support – for this, use something firm but not hard.
- Move the patient every few hours to relieve pressure areas.

Modified recovery position (for suspected spinal injury)

Extend the arm closest to you straight above the casualty's head. Log roll the casualty onto one side, and rest the head on the extended arm. Either keep the legs straight or bend them to improve stability. Support in place with sleeping bags, bedding, sails, or similar. Turn the casualty every few hours to prevent pressure sores.

Log roll

Always use a log roll if you suspect there is a spinal injury. Other reasons include:
- To inspect the back of the casualty for injuries
- To place the casualty in a modified recovery position while waiting to evacuate
- To manoeuvre a recovery stretcher underneath the casualty

It takes a minimum of three people to log roll (do your best if you only have two – *see* illustration below). Ideally, there will be four, so the fourth can examine. The aim of the log roll is to keep the entire spine in one line (not just the neck). Fit a semi-rigid collar to the neck before rolling if possible, to protect the cervical spine (*see* p.164).

Method
- Position yourselves as illustrated below, kneeling and stable.
- The first person keeps control and immobilizes the cervical spine, with or without a semi-rigid collar. This person controls all movements and must be very clear in giving instructions to the others.
- The second person puts one hand on the casualty's shoulder and one hand on the top of the thigh.
- The third person puts one hand on the top of the pelvis, above the lower hand of the second person, and the other hand on the lower leg, just below the knee.
- On the command of the first person, smoothly rotate the casualty by 90°, to come to rest against the knees of person two and person three.
- Hold the casualty in that position until the examination is complete or the spinal board/stretcher is in place.
- On the command of the first person, smoothly rotate the casualty back into the original position.

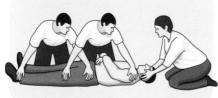

Log roll technique with three people: one person stabilizes the neck.

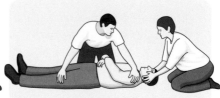

Log roll technique with two people: a third may examine the back.

Notes
- Performing a log roll on a casualty in a bunk is not easy. Use the principles above, but modify as necessary. It is important to leave the casualty facing outwards, so you can see the face and assess for breathing, vomit, and secretions.
- If only three people can help, two may need to log roll while the third examines.

SPINAL IMMOBILIZATION

Immobilization of the cervical spine involves fitting a semi-rigid collar to the neck with side blocks and then strapping the casualty to a long spinal board. Only then is the entire spine fully immobilized and protected from further damage.

Indications for immobilizing the spine

- Obvious head or neck trauma
- Injury to the upper chest
- Injury to another part of the spine
- Numbness or tingling in the arms or legs following an accident
- An accident of strong force, such as collision with the boom causing LoC or a 3m fall from the rig
- Trauma involving multiple injuries
- Injury to the pelvis

> If in doubt, immobilize the casualty with a semi-rigid collar and spinal board.

Fitting a semi-rigid collar

Maintain manual immobilization of the cervical spine while the collar is being fitted (**1**); keep this up until the casualty is fully immobilized on a spinal board or something similar.

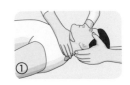

Method

- In finger widths, measure the distance between the jaw line and top of shoulders. Match this height with the hard-plastic part of the collar that fits over the shoulder, beneath the ear. Collars come in a variety of sizes, or are adjustable, and should come with sizing instructions.
- Slide the back of the collar under the neck all the way through to the other side (**2**).

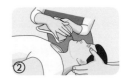

- Rotate the front part over the neck, making sure the chin rest fits snugly under the chin, lifting it somewhat, so that the head is tilted back slightly (**3**).
- Fasten hook-and-loop tape firmly to the back of the collar (**4**).

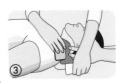

- If the casualty is conscious, check that the collar is comfortable. It should fit securely around the neck, but should not be tight and should not impede breathing.
- If the casualty is unconscious, try to fit your finger between the casualty's skin and the collar; you should be able to do this without too much difficulty.

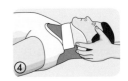

Notes

- Semi-rigid collars can cause pressure sores if left on for too long. Remove the collar for a few minutes every two hours until the casualty is evacuated.
- A collar can be improvised by wrapping a tightly rolled towel around the neck, under the chin, and taping it in position.

Immobilizing a casualty on a spinal board

- Remember to immobilize the cervical spine first, using either a purpose-designed, semi-rigid collar or an improvised collar, such as a rolled towel.
- After stabilizing the cervical spine, ABCDE assessment (*see* p.32) takes priority over placing the casualty onto a spinal board.
- Once these actions are completed, move the casualty onto the spinal board as soon as you can. Keep the casualty in this position for a maximum of 2 hours only, to avoid pressure sore formation.

Method

- Log roll the casualty onto one side (*see* p.163).
- Place the spinal board snugly under the casualty as far as it will go, without moving the casualty.
- Smoothly rotate the casualty until they are facing upwards on the board.
- If you need to slide the casualty further onto the board: keep the cervical spine immobilized, and on command, gently slide the casualty, keeping the spine in line, until the body lies squarely on the board.

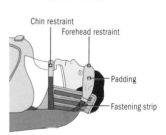

- Maintaining cervical spine immobilization, secure straps in these positions:
  - Around the upper chest, including the arms
  - Around the pelvis, including the arms
  - Around the thighs
  - Around the calves

Full spinal immobilization

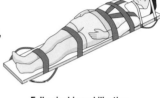

Chin restraint
Forehead restraint
Padding
Fastening strip

- Make sure the straps are firm but not too tight, so they don't impede breathing.
- Secure the head and collar to the board.
- Fix padded blocks or rolled towels on either side of the head.
- Fix straps over the forehead and over the front part of the collar.

Immobilizing the head and neck on a spinal board

- When this process is completed, manual immobilization can cease and the casualty can be transported on the board.

Notes

- Beware vomiting, because the casualty cannot move. If vomiting does occur, turn the board on its side immediately to prevent vomit from entering the lungs.
- Being immobilized may cause feelings of claustrophobia and the casualty may struggle, especially if confused. Small amounts of diazepam may be required (2mg intravenously every 30 minutes as needed), but seek medical advice first. Be very careful about sedating a brain-injured casualty.
- A spinal board can be improvised from a long storm board and sail ties. Use a foam mat or sleeping bag under the casualty to reduce pressure points.
- The casualty should only stay on a spinal board for a maximum of two hours before being transfered to a firm mattress – a bunk mattress will usually have to suffice.

PULSE AND BLOOD PRESSURE

There are a number of ways to assess how a person's heart – more accurately, their cardiovascular system – is performing. Pulse and blood pressure are basic vital signs, and it is essential to know how to measure them accurately.

General appearance A casualty who is sick tends to look pale and will have cold hands and feet. A casualty who has had a cardiac arrest will look white.

Pulse In a patient who is unwell, the pulse may be very slow (<45 beats per minute) or very fast (>130 beats per minute).

Blood pressure Check the blood pressure, which may be low (<90mmHg systolic pressure) or very high (>160mmHg).

Perfusion of the skin Assess blood flow to the skin, which may be reduced (capillary refill time >4 seconds – *see* opposite page).

Measuring the pulse

☐ The pulse can be felt anywhere in the body where an artery lies close to the skin.

☐ Feel for the pulse firmly with two fingers but not too hard or you may block off the blood supply.

☐ Use a watch or a clock with a second hand and count for 30 seconds.

☐ Don't estimate a rate – you could be significantly wrong, which may adversely affect treatment.

IN AN EMERGENCY

Measure the carotid pulse
Feel for the pulse in the groove between the larynx (voice box) and the muscles of the neck.

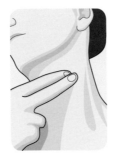

Measure the femoral pulse
Feel for the pulse in the skin groove in the groin, at the top of the leg.

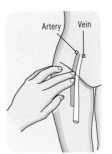

IN A ROUTINE CHECK

Measure the radial pulse
Feel for the pulse at the wrist about 3cm above the base of the thumb.

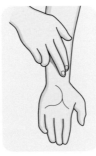

Measure the brachial pulse
Feel for the pulse at the elbow, on the inside edge of the bicep.

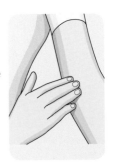

Measuring blood pressure

The blood pressure has two values. In the example 120/70mmHg:

Systolic blood pressure (SBP) – is the higher value (120mmHg).
Diastolic blood pressure (DBP) – is the lower value (70mmHg).

Method

☐ Position the casualty in a seated position or lying down if necessary.
☐ Fasten the cuff around the upper arm. Larger people need larger cuffs.
☐ Pump the cuff while taking the radial pulse. Make sure you can feel a clear pulse before you begin to pump.
☐ Note the pressure on the dial (in mmHg) when you lose the pulse. Inflate the cuff another 20–30mmHg and then very slowly, still feeling the pulse, let the air out of the cuff with the screw valve.

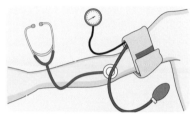

☐ The pressure at which the pulse reappears is the SBP.
☐ Inflate the cuff to 20–30mmHg above the SBP, and listen with a stethoscope over the brachial artery. Let the air out slowly.

Inflatable cuff and bulb, stethoscope, and measurement dial.

☐ At about the SBP, you will hear a tapping noise made by the pulse reappearing in the brachial artery.
☐ Continue to let the air out of the cuff slowly, listening to the tapping noise. When the tapping disappears, note the pressure. This is the DBP.

Estimating the blood pressure

It may not be possible to measure the blood pressure by the technique above. You can estimate the SBP by feeling various pulses (*see* opposite page for locations):

If a radial pulse is present: SBP >70mmHg
If a brachial pulse is present: SBP >60mmHg
If a carotid pulse is present: SBP >50mmHg

These are only estimates. Look at the patient as a whole.

Automated blood pressure measurement

Many medical kits contain an automated blood pressure measuring device. Most of these will be self-explanatory, but instructions should be supplied. It may be difficult to take a reading if the blood pressure is very low or if there is an irregular pulse.

Capillary refill time (CRT)

This is a method for assessing skin perfusion, which indicates the degree of shock and tests the blood supply. If the casualty is very cold, this may cause a longer CRT.

☐ Press on the fleshy part at the end of a finger (or forehead) for 4 seconds.
☐ Release and time how long it takes for the white "blanch" mark to pink up again.
☐ This should take less than 2 seconds. A CRT longer than 4 seconds indicates that the casualty may require IV fluids (*see* p.172).

ASSESSING CONSCIOUS STATE: GLASGOW COMA SCALE (GCS) AND AVPU

The conscious state of the sick or injured casualty may vary from being completely awake and alert to being deeply unconscious and unrousable.

AVPU and GCS are ways of assessing the conscious state and giving it a value. Repeating the measurement over time allows you to detect deterioration or improvement in the level of consciousness and take appropriate action. AVPU is a simplified, fast system for scoring the conscious state. GCS is a more comprehensive and sensitive method but takes more skill and time. A small deterioration in conscious state is easier to spot when using the GCS scale.

AVPU

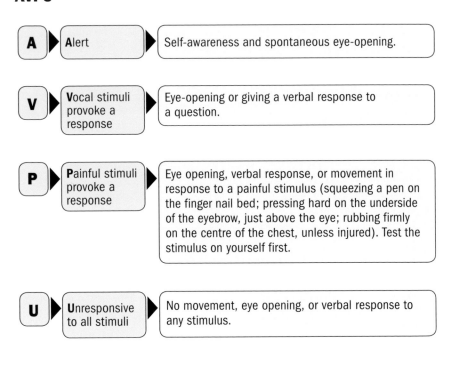

A ▶ **A**lert ▶ Self-awareness and spontaneous eye-opening.

V ▶ **V**ocal stimuli provoke a response ▶ Eye-opening or giving a verbal response to a question.

P ▶ **P**ainful stimuli provoke a response ▶ Eye opening, verbal response, or movement in response to a painful stimulus (squeezing a pen on the finger nail bed; pressing hard on the underside of the eyebrow, just above the eye; rubbing firmly on the centre of the chest, unless injured). Test the stimulus on yourself first.

U ▶ **U**nresponsive to all stimuli ▶ No movement, eye opening, or verbal response to any stimulus.

Document the time and conscious level

Glasgow Coma Scale

- GCS measures the combination of eye, motor, and verbal responses to stimulation.
- The response that should be recorded is the best one the casualty gives. That means, if the casualty has an injured arm which cannot move, but can move the other one, that response should be counted.
- Poking the tongue out or opening or closing the eyes on request counts as obeying a command.
- Speaking clearly in a foreign language counts as talking normally, even if you cannot understand.

	Best Response	Score
Eyes	Eyes open spontaneously	4
	Eyes open on being asked a question	3
	Eyes open on painful stimulus	2
	Eyes stay shut	1
Motor	Obeys commands (squeezes hands, pokes tongue out)	6
	Moves hand to stop painful stimulus (localizes)	5
	Withdraws hand/arm or leg from painful stimulus	4
	Bends up arms and legs to painful stimulus	3
	Straightens arms and legs to painful stimulus	2
	No movement of any part of the body to any stimulus	1
Verbal	Gives answers to questions, seems orientated	5
	Answers questions but shows confusion	4
	Speaks in single words, no sentences	3
	Makes incomprehensible sounds	2
	Gives no verbal response	1
The maximum GCS Is 15	Fully awake and not confused	
The minimum GCS is 3	Deeply unconscious and unresponsive	

Notes
- A GCS of 8 or less implies the casualty may not be able to maintain their own airway. They may inhale vomit or secretions into the lungs, or the tongue may obstruct the airway and prevent breathing. Put the casualty into the recovery position (see pp.162–163).
- Make sure injuries are not intefering with the assessment: limbs may be paralysed; swelling may prevent the eyes from opening; and mouth injuries may impede speech.
- A change of 2 or more in the GCS implies a significant change in conscious level.

> ## Document the time and the total score
> Also note the scores for each separate response

REHYDRATION

The body normally controls its own level of hydration. However, trauma and illness can upset this balance. In hospital, sterile intravenous (IV) fluid can usually be infused directly into a casualty's circulation through a cannula, which is inserted into a vein. On a boat, however, the equipment and expertise required for giving IV fluids may not always be available.

Alternative rehydration methods include the oral route, a nasogastric tube, and, if other methods are not possible, the rectal route. Sterile intravenous fluid can be used for all three methods.

Oral route Giving fluids by mouth is the most effective and convenient way of achieving hydration. The fluid should be clean, but does not have to be sterile. DO NOT USE WATER ALONE if severe diarrhoea, vomiting, and/or sweating occurs. Instead, give a solution that will replace lost chemicals (see opposite page). DO NOT USE THE ORAL ROUTE if the casualty is not fully conscious – vomit may enter the lungs. If the casualty is awake and vomiting only occasionally, it may be worth persisting with oral fluids. Administer antinausea drugs to prevent vomiting.

Nasogastric (NG) tube (see p.186) An NG tube can be used in an unconscious casualty but not if they are vomiting. Give antinausea medication (see pp.208–211). NG tubes are not easy to insert, so seek prior medical advice.

Rectal route (see p.188) If intractable vomiting occurs or if IV access is impossible, the rectal route may be the only option. This can be effective, but fluid absorption will be limited.

Routine fluid losses per day for a typical 70kg crew

Route of loss	Amount lost per day (ml)
☐ Perspiration (no work)	700
☐ Breath	500
☐ Urine	1300
☐ Faeces	100
TOTAL	**2600ml/day**

Note Losses due to perspiration (particularly in hot climates and with physical exertion) may increase to above 5000ml.

Daily fluid requirements

For the average-sized man: 3000ml/day
For the average-sized woman: 2200ml/day

These amounts fulfil the body's normal daily requirements. See the opposite page for guidance on giving extra fluid.

Reasons for emergency rehydration

- Severe vomiting
- Profuse diarrhoea
- Blood loss
- Severe heat illness
- Burns
- Diabetic crisis
- Hydration for unconscious casualty
- Shock (other causes)

Emergency rehydration

The amount of fluid you give will be guided by specific circumstances.

Immediately Give 500ml of fluid by the easiest route available (IV if unconscious).

Assess Check level of hydration/shock (*see* below).

Check medical history If the casualty has a heart, lung, or kidney disease, seek medical advice before giving more than 1L of fluid.

Continue giving fluid until signs of shock reduce If the casualty still looks shocked after being given 1.5L of fluid, seek medical advice for guidance.

Maintain daily requirements Give fluids until casualty is drinking well or evacuated.

Estimating and replacing blood loss

- Estimating blood loss is difficult. Estimate in 250ml amounts (approximately one cup) – for example, blood loss may be estimated at 250ml, 500ml, or 750ml.
- For every **1000ml blood loss**, the casualty requires **3000ml fluid replacement** with a clear crystalloid solution (e.g. Ringer's Lactate or 0.9% normal saline solution).
- If you use colloid solutions (e.g. gelatin or albumin solutions), give the 1000ml solution per 1000ml of blood loss at first and reassess. The casualty will probably need more.

Assessing level of hydration

Signs of continued dehydration include:

- Fast pulse rate (>100bpm)
- Low blood pressure
- Pale/white skin
- Cold skin on distal arms and legs
- Dark urine (should be pale or colourless)
- Urine output less than 30ml/hour for average-sized adult

Giving more fluid (500ml at a time) should reverse these signs.

Emergency mixture for oral/NG/rectal fluid rehydration

Use premade oral rehydration salts (ORS) such as those produced by the World Health Organization. Alternate 1L ORS and then 1L water, as required.

OR

Emergency ORS solution:

- 1L clean water
- Add 6 level teaspoons of sugar (or 2 teaspoons of honey)
- Add ½ level teaspoon of table salt
- Add a generous squeeze of lemon/orange/lime/grapefruit juice or a spoonful of mashed banana
- Taste the mixture yourself first: it should be slightly salty.

VENOUS AND INTRAOSSEOUS ACCESS

IV route

The venous route is very effective for giving both fluids and drugs. They are delivered directly into the circulation and can begin to work immediately. However, inserting a cannula requires training, and regular practice should be undertaken to maintain the skill. There are risks involved in using a cannula (see below), so observe good hygiene and wear gloves.

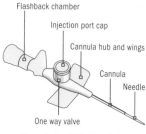

Cannula for IV fluid and drugs

Inserting a cannula

Method for inserting a cannula

□ Fix a tourniquet firmly around the upper arm (**1**).If necessary, someone can put their hands around the arm to act as a tourniquet.

□ Wait for a few minutes for the veins to appear.
  - Ask the casualty to clench and unclench the hand.
  - Tap the veins, which will make them expand.
  - Hang the arm down the side of the bed or bunk, and let blood run into the arm.

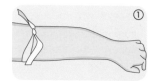

□ Clean the skin over a suitable vein with an antiseptic swab or solution.

□ Using two fingers, gently stretch the skin on either side of the vein and pull it towards you (**2**).

□ Line the cannula up with the vein, at an angle of about 30° to the skin.

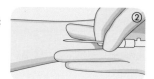

□ Insert the tip of the cannula through the skin, and then reduce the angle to about 15° (**3**).

□ Advance slowly into the vein. Watch the back end of the cannula very carefully and stop advancing immediately when you see a flash of blood.

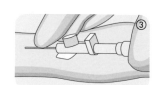

□ Hold the back end of the needle very still and advance the wings or hub of the cannula so the plastic tube goes into the vein. The tube should advance easily. If not, start again.

□ Release the tourniquet.

□ Take the stopper off the back end of the needle and screw it to the end of the cannula (**4**).

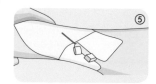

□ Fix the cannula securely in place with a cannula-fixing dressing or with purpose-designed tape (**5**).

□ Flush the cannula with a 5ml syringe of normal saline - this should not cause any swelling or pain.

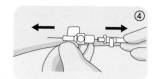

Cautions and complications

- ☐ Larger cannulas allow greater fluid flow but are more difficult to put in.
- ☐ Only use sterile fluid that is intended (licensed) for IV use.
- ☐ Be very careful that no air enters the cannula – may cause cardiac arrest or stroke.
- ☐ Watch for infection: redness of the skin; pain on injection; swelling; blockage. If any of these signs occur, remove the cannula.
- ☐ The cannula can stay in place for 5 days, unless it becomes infected, painful, or blocked. If it does, remove it earlier and insert a new one in a different place.

Sites for inserting a cannula

- ☐ Back of hand: good for normal IV fluids and drugs
- ☐ Wrist: good for resuscitating fluids and larger cannulas
- ☐ Inside of the elbow: larger veins make it easier to get a cannula in, but the arm must stay straight
- ☐ Feet/lower leg: can also be considered.

Intraosseous (IO) access

If you can't get IV access in an emergency, consider IO access, which allows fast fluid replacement through an IO needle (1L every 30 minutes), and administration of adrenaline and other drugs. This method involves inserting a needle directly into the bone – usually just below the knee on the inside of the tibia (shin bone) – and can be used for several hours before being replaced with IV access. IO access requires a special hollow needle with a trocar. There are also specialized devices that "fire" or drill the needle into the bone. DO NOT USE in a leg with a suspected fracture, infected skin, an open wound, infected bone, or known osteoporosis.

Method for gaining IO access

- ☐ Wear sterile gloves and clean the skin with antiseptic cleansing solution.
- ☐ Identify the site for needle insertion (**1**): on the flat of the inside of the shin bone, about 5cm below the knee (in an average sized adult).
- ☐ Support the leg behind the knee, which should be slightly bent.
- ☐ Firmly insert the needle (or drill or "fire" the device, holding it firmly) through the skin at right angles (**2**).
- ☐ Advance the needle into the bone, twisting it, until you feel a "give" – may be subtle.
- ☐ The needle should remain upright in the bone by itself. Remove trocar (**3**).
- ☐ Flush the needle with 5ml normal saline, which should go in easily.
- ☐ Connect the infusion line and tape to the leg (**4**).

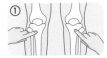 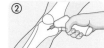 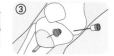 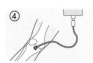

Cautions and complications

- ☐ The leg may swell either around the needle or generally. This means the needle is inserted incorrectly – stop the infusion and take it out.
- ☐ Infection may affect skin or bone. Watch for redness, swelling, and pain. If these signs develop, remove the needle and treat with antibiotics.

INJECTIONS AND INFUSIONS

Injections may be given into a vein (intravenously), into a muscle (intramuscularly), or under the skin (subcutaneously), using a syringe and needle. Not all injectable drugs can be given in all three ways, so read the individual drug instructions or seek medical advice.

An infusion is a means of injecting fluid into a vein continually over hours or even days via a cannula. This process involves special tubing (known as a "giving set") and sterile fluid specifically designed for infusion into the vein.

General rules

☐ Make sure you have the correct drug in the appropriate dosage for the casualty. Ask somebody else to double check. It is very easy to make a mistake.
☐ Keep the procedure sterile: clean the skin before injecting with an alcohol wipe designed for the purpose or a cotton swab soaked in chlorhexadine and ensure that the end of the syringe or needle does not become contaminated.
☐ When drawing up the drug, make sure there is no air in the syringe. To expel any air, hold the syringe needle upwards and slowly push the plunger in.
☐ Check the casualty afterwards for signs of an allergic reaction (see pp.50–51).
☐ Dispose of all needles and other sharp objects safely, to avoid injuries.

IV injections

The best veins for IV injections are on the insides of the elbows, but look for others if you can't find these.

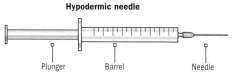

Hypodermic needle

Plunger   Barrel   Needle

☐ Prepare the drug and clean the skin.

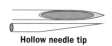

Hollow needle tip

☐ Put a tourniquet around the upper arm, and let the arm hang down to fill the veins with blood.
☐ Put a finger either side of the vein where you want to inject, and pull the skin apart and towards you.
☐ Insert the needle, hole upwards, at an angle of 30° to the skin (**1**), pointing up the arm (towards the heart) (**2**). Once the tip is inside the skin, pull back on the plunger slightly.

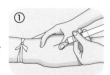

☐ When the tip of the needle enters the vein, blood will appear in the syringe barrel. Stop advancing the needle. Release the tourniquet before injecting.
☐ Inject the drug slowly and smoothly, checking for any swelling around the tip of the needle. If there is swelling, the tip is not in the vein, so start again.

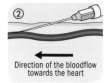

Direction of the bloodflow towards the heart

☐ When you are finished, smoothly remove the needle from the skin, press down firmly on the injection site with a cotton swab for a few minutes, then apply an adhesive bandage.

Intramuscular injections

Intramuscular (IM) injections are easier than IV ones. DO NOT give IM shot if the casualty takes anticoagulants – will bleed.

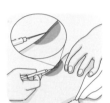

□ The two main sites for giving an IM injection are the shoulder (**1**) and the outer, upper side of the buttock (**2**).

□ Use a green (size 21 gauge) needle for an average-sized adult and use a blue (23 gauge) needle for a small adult.

□ Clean the skin over the injection site.

□ Hold the syringe firmly by the barrel like a dart, and aim it at 90° to the skin.

□ In one smooth movement, push the entire needle in.

□ Pull back on the plunger. If blood appears in the syringe barrel, the needle is in a blood vessel. Withdraw it 5mm, angle the needle to one side, and push it in again. Repeat until you are certain that the needle is not in a blood vessel.

□ Inject the plunger smoothly over 5 seconds.

□ Withdraw the needle and press on the site with a cotton swab.

Subcutaneous injections

Subcutaneous injections are similar to IM injections but not as deep. Follow the same rules for preparation. Absorption of the drug may be very slow if the casualty is cold and the blood supply to the skin is limited.

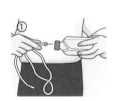

□ Use an orange (25 gauge) needle.

□ Pinch the skin on the shoulder gently between your thumb and forefinger, pulling up a ridge of skin.

Inject under the skin at a low angle.

□ Push the needle into the skin on the top of the ridge at a low angle, to about half the length of the needle; smoothly inject over a few seconds.

□ Withdraw the needle and press on the site with a cotton swab.

Setting up an infusion

This is a sterile procedure so avoid touching the connectors.

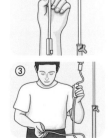

□ The giving set has a roller valve. Turn this off before you begin.

□ The giving set has a sharp, piercing end which should be inserted into the special port on the bag or bottle of fluid (**1**).

□ Hang the bag or bottle upside down, and squeeze the drip chamber until it is half full of fluid (**2**).

□ Open the roller valve and watch the fluid flow down the tubing to the end. Keep flushing through until all the air bubbles have gone. Shut off the roller valve.

□ Connect the tubing to the cannula, sited in the vein.

□ Open the roller valve and adjust the drip rate to give the desired flow (**3**).

□ Tape the tubing to the arm twice to ensure the cannula stays in place.

MINOR OPERATIVE SET-UP

Conditions on a vessel may make it more difficult to achieve a sterile environment for the occasional minor medical procedure. However, good preparation will improve the outcome.

Procedures that might require operative set-up
☐ Wound repair (cleaning, suturing/stapling, dressing)
☐ Incising, draining, and wicking an abscess
☐ Inserting a chest drain
☐ Inserting a urinary catheter
☐ Inserting a rectal rehydration tube
☐ Inserting an IV cannula
☐ Performing a nerve block
☐ Cleaning, reducing, and dressing an open fracture

Preparing the casualty
☐ Explain exactly what you are going to do. Be truthful about whether the procedure will be painful.
☐ Find a comfortable and stable position and try to put the casualty at ease: administer adequate pain relief (local anaesthesia and longer acting analgesia); maintain privacy and dignity (do not make jokes); and keep the casualty warm.
☐ Notwithstanding privacy and warmth, it is important to get good exposure of the area you are going to be dealing with. If anything, expose more of the body than you need to, so you don't have to make adjustments while you are wearing sterile gloves.
☐ When everything is ready, you will need to clean a good area around the site with a sterilizing skin preparation fluid. Make sure the casualty is not allergic to the sterilizing fluid.

Preparing yourself
☐ Ask for medical advice before you start, not during or after the procedure.
☐ Make sure you will have a comfortable and stable working position. This depends on the state of the casualty, but two options are: sitting together at the navigation table; sitting at the galley table, with the casualty lying on it. You may operate on a sick casualty in a bunk, but this position is slightly restricted.
☐ If you are even slightly seasick, take some antinausea drugs before you start.
☐ Make sure your arms are bare to above the elbow, and wash thoroughly with soap and water. If there is pure alcohol or chlorhexadine on board, you can use it to sterilize your hands.
☐ Recruit somebody to help in case you need it, and don't be afraid to ask.
☐ When you are ready, put on a sterile pair of gloves that fit you. If there are no sterile gloves on board, wear nonsterile gloves, and rub your gloved hands in sterilizing skin preparation fluid.

Preparing the boat

- Always perform medical procedures during quiet periods on deck (when you are not close to land or surrounded by shipping, for example) unless very urgent.
- Turn the boat downwind if there is any kind of sea running. It will make a considerable difference to stability.
- Avoid any dramatic manoeuvres with the boat.
- Make sure the person on the helm is experienced and trustworthy.
- Make sure the operative site is as well lit as possible – head torches work well.

Preparing the equipment

- Gather all the equipment you might need before you begin.
- Instruments can be sterilized by boiling them for twenty minutes and then allowing them to cool, or by washing them in sterilizing skin preparation fluid if nothing else is available. Some medical kits include specific instrument-sterilizing fluid or sterile procedure packs, which contain a range of sterile equipment.

- You may need:
  - Sterile forceps
  - Sterile scissors
  - Sutures or staples and stapler
  - Disposable razor (for removing hair)
  - Sterile skin drape for around the site
  - Sterile pot for fluid
  - Sterile haemostatic clamp
  - Sterile scalpel
  - Sterile swabs
  - Sterilizing skin preperation fluid
  - Sterile drape for set-up
  - Sterile tweezers

- Use one sterile drape to make a sterile field, where you can place all equipment.
- Make sure you choose a stable area, so the equipment doesn't fall onto the floor if the boat rolls.

Minor operative set-up

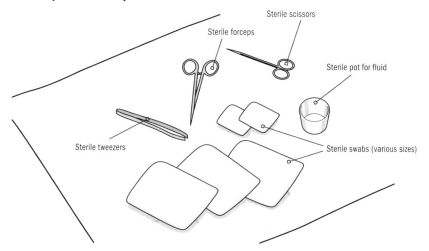

Sterile scissors

Sterile forceps

Sterile pot for fluid

Sterile tweezers

Sterile swabs (various sizes)

REPAIRING THE SKIN

A deep and gaping wound that is left open to heal by itself will leave a large scar, whereas a wound that is neatly closed, using one of the methods described below, will heal leaving a small scar. Always use sterile gloves and prepare a sterile field.

Wounds that should NOT be closed

- Gaping wounds, with substantial tissue loss and edges that will not join easily
- Wounds that have been become infected (pus in the wound)
- Wounds that have been open for longer than 18 hours
- Wounds that are contaminated and cannot be properly cleaned, which are likely to become infected. Any sutures will need to be removed to allow pus to discharge.

These wounds should be cleaned gently but as thoroughly as possible and then dressed with sterile gauze and bandaging. The wound should be inspected each day and cleaned with sterile fluid. If it looks infected, start oral antibiotics.

Methods for repairing skin wounds

Method	Difficulty	Indications	Cautions
Adhesive wound closure strips	Easy	Small incisions less than 10cm long	Not good in the damp or over joints
Skin staples	Difficult	Wounds on the trunk, scalp, arms, and legs	Do not use on face and neck
Tissue adhesive (skin glue)	Moderate	Small incisions less than 10cm in length; clean edges	Do not use in the damp or over joints; do not get in the eye
Sutures	Difficult	Large, ragged wounds; wounds in skin over joints; persistent bleeding	Use thinner thread on the face, lips (see below)

Adhesive wound closure strips

- Make sure the wound has stopped bleeding and is completely dry and clean.
- Starting at one end, gently use an adhesive strip to pull the edges of the wound together and then stick down the other side (**1**); if the edges are jagged, bring together matching parts and stick them in place.

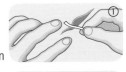

- Move to the next point, 5mm from the first. Depending on how many strips are available, stick two strips parallel to the wound, one on either side (**2**).

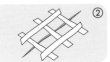

- Place a dressing over the wound to keep it dry and clean.
- Leave the strips on until they fall off. Some may need replacing before the wound has healed properly.
- Skin glue can be used to stick strips more firmly.

Skin staples

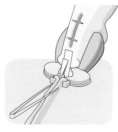

- Position the skin edges together with the cut edges pointing to the outside. This will prevent outer skin from being stapled inside the wound.
- With the edges in place, position the stapler as shown (right) and staple the skin. Insert staples 5mm apart.
- If the wound has jagged edges, staple matching pieces in several places, then staple from one end.
- Place a sterile dressing over the wound.

Use a pair of forceps to hold the wound edges together.

- Leave the staples for as long as you would sutures (*see* below). Inspect regularly for infection and swelling. You may need to remove staples to let pus out.

Skin glue

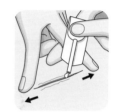

- Use on straight, dry, nonbleeding cuts, not over joints.
- Hold skin together and run glue along the wound edges.
- Do not get glue inside the cut – tissue will not heal.
- Apply up to three layers (see product instructions).
- Hold edges together for 30 seconds. Full bond should develop in 2–3 minutes.
- Usually no dressing is needed, but keep the wound dry.
- The adhesive should come off naturally after 7–10 days.

Apply skin glue on either side of the wound.

Sutures (silk, polyester, or polyamide – thread bonded to a needle)

- Use local anaesthetic (up to 10ml 2% lidocaine) if putting in more than 2 sutures.
- Begin by putting a suture in halfway along the wound, then in each quarter, then fill in the gaps, leaving about 5mm between sutures.
- If the wound has jagged edges, match these up first and suture them in place.
- Use "interrupted" sutures as in (**1**). Hold the skin edges up with a pair of forceps (the toothed kind work well) while you put the needle in approximately 5mm from the wound edge and curve it deeply into the skin (**2**), then through the opposite edge (**3**); aim to exit 5mm from the wound on the other side.
- Tie with a reef knot (**4**), pulling the knot just tightly enough to bring the skin edges together and no tighter, or lack of blood flow will prevent healing.
- If you are not satisfied with a suture, take it out and start again.
- Clean the wound and apply a sterile dressing.
- Inspect every two days. If the wound looks red and swollen, release a suture and see if pus comes out. Leave the suture out and reapply a fresh dressing.

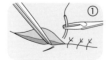   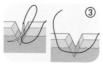 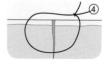

When to remove sutures and clips

- Face: 3–5 days
- Scalp: 7–10 days
- Limbs: 10–14 days
- Joints: 14 days
- Trunk: 7–10 days

CHEST DRAINS AND EMERGENCY CHEST DECOMPRESSION

A tension pneumothorax (see pp.88–89) is rare on a boat, but may occur. Prompt action to release the pressure build-up inside the chest may prevent collapse. Once the chest has been decompressed with a needle, insert a chest drain (or adapt a urinary catheter to use as a chest drain). Chest seal dressings, incorporating a one-way valve, are also available.

An emergency chest decompression may be required for a suspected tension pneumothorax: seek medical advice at once and arrange urgent evacuation. Suspected blood in the chest cavity (haemothorax – see p.89) should not require emergency decompression, but does require IV cannulation and fluids for resuscitation. In all cases, seek urgent medical advice.

Signs of a tension pneumothorax	Signs of a haemothorax
□ Difficulty in breathing □ Low blood pressure □ The trachea may be shifted away from the side of the chest with the air in it □ Reduced breath sounds on the side of the chest with the air in it	□ Difficulty in breathing □ Casualty may be shocked (low blood pressure) □ Reduced breath sounds on the side of the chest with the blood in it

Emergency chest decompression

Decompression involves inserting a cannula into the front of the chest on the side where you suspect there may be a tension pneumothorax.

□ Position the casualty in a stable position, sitting up at 30° if possible.

□ Use sterile gloves and a sterile field (see pp.176–77).

□ Use a 14- or 16-gauge cannula (the larger the better).

□ Locate the position to insert the cannula: draw an imaginary line down the chest from the midpoint of the collar bone; locate the second space between the ribs along this line. This should be approximately 5–8cm below the collar bone in an adult.

□ Clean the area and inject local anaesthetic under the skin (2.5–5ml 2% lidocaine if available).

□ Insert the cannula at 90° to the skin, up to the hilt. Remove any stopper from the end of the cannula before inserting.

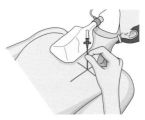

Draw lines to mark a clear insertion point for the cannula.

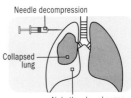

Needle decompression

Collapsed lung

Air in the pleural space

Interior view: decompression for tension pneumothorax

- If there is air under pressure in the pleural space, you will hear a hiss when the tip of the needle penetrates.
- Leave the cannula and needle in position. Only remove them if a chest drain is inserted.
- If blood comes out instead of air, leave the cannula where it is, seek medical advice, and consider inserting a chest drain.
- It is possible to fit a flutter valve on the end of the cannula (see p.182).
- The cannula can be taped upright, surrounded by gauze, to protect it from being dislodged (do not bend the cannula over so it is parallel with the skin).
- Monitor the casualty, including vital signs, to check for improvement.
- If the casualty does not improve, seek urgent medical advice, and consider repeating the procedure one rib space lower.

Inserting a chest drain (Seldinger technique)

Placing a chest drain involves putting a larger tube through the side of the chest into the pleural space. This is a more invasive procedure than chest decompression with a needle, and ideally should be performed with a specific chest drain kit. Always seek medical advice before attempting this procedure.

- Insert an IV line before you start, in case there is an emergency.
- Position the casualty sitting up at 30° if possible, in a stable position.
- Use sterile gloves and prepare a sterile field (see pp.176–77).
- Locate the correct insertion point: on an imaginary line down the chest from the middle of the armpit in the "safe triangle" (1), between the pectoralis major (chest muscle) and the latissimus dorsi (the main muscle at the side of the back), above the level of the nipple (see diagram).

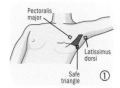

- Clean the area and inject local anaesthetic into the skin (10ml 1% lidocaine if available).
- Insert the cannula just over the top of the lower rib, angling the needle slightly towards the feet, pulling back gently on the syringe as you go.

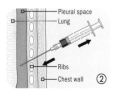

- Once air or blood is aspirated, stop advancing the needle, and push the plastic cannula around the outside of the needle, into the chest.
- Advance the cannula smoothly to its hub, withdraw the needle, fasten the syringe onto the cannula, and pull back on the syringe. You should suck air or blood into the barrel (2). If you don't, start again. If after three attempts you are still unsuccessful, stop and seek medical advice.

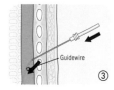

- When you are satisfied the cannula is in the right place, insert the guidewire from the holder through the cannula and into the chest, leaving about 15cm free (3). Keep hold of it.

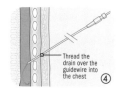

□ Remove the cannula, and thread the dilator over the wire through the chest wall, using a twisting motion. You may need to make a small cut in the skin with a scalpel to ease the way in (**4**). If there is more than one dilator, start with the smallest and work up sequentially. Keep a firm hold on the wire throughout.

□ When the last dilator is in place, thread the chest drain tube onto the dilator and insert it, in a similar manner, into the chest, to a depth of 15–20cm, depending on the drain and the size of the casualty.

□ Remove the wire, and attach the tubing to a flutter valve (*see* below).

□ Insert two sutures at the entry site and tie very firmly around the chest drain tube, but not so tightly that the tube is obstructed.

□ Stick the tube to the chest with plenty of tape so it doesn't get dislodged.

□ Place a sterile dressing over the insertion site and inspect each day.

□ Monitor the casualty and vital signs, checking for improvement.

□ If there is no improvement, seek urgent medical advice.

□ Arrange to evacuate the casualty urgently.

One-way valves for chest drains or open chest wounds

In hospitals, underwater seals are usually used as one-way valves, to allow air out of the chest but not back in. This method is impracticable on a boat and could be dangerous. A flutter valve is a better option; either from the kit or improvised.

Heimlich flutter valve

□ This is a simple, plastic flutter valve within a clear plastic casing.

□ The valve fastens to the tubing from the chest drain and then another tube leads from the valve to a drainage bag (you could improvise with a urine drainage bag).

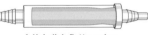

A Heimlich flutter valve may be included in the boat's medical kit.

□ Make sure you connect the valve the right way round.

Chest seal dressing

□ These incorporate a one-way valve which lets air and fluid out of the chest, but not back in.

□ Apply firmly over the chest wound and follow the instructions on the packet.

□ Monitor casualty and seek medical advice immediately.

Flutter valve for an open chest wound

□ Soak a gauze dressing swab in petroleum jelly.

□ After cleaning the wound with sterilizing fluid, place the dressing over the hole, and tape it firmly on three sides, leaving the fourth side open.

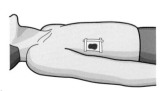

□ This flap acts as a valve, letting air out but not back in again.

□ Consider inserting a chest drain through the wound, but seek medical advice first.

Leave one side of the dressing open to act as a flutter valve.

INCISION AND DRAINAGE OF AN ABSCESS

On a boat, abscesses commonly form in haematomas (bruises), which become infected: these are relatively easy to open and drain. Abscesses that form elsewhere (on the buttocks, breasts, or perianal area) may be more deep-seated, requiring a more invasive approach. In such cases, seek medical advice.

Small, superficial abscesses (<5mm in diameter)

☐ Use a hot compress to encourage the abscess to "point" (towards the surface).
☐ The abscess may then self-discharge – a compress with magnesium sulphate paste may help.
☐ Apply a sterile dressing.

Larger abscesses near the skin surface

☐ Position the casualty in a comfortable position, and explain what you are going to do. Local anaesthetic does not work well around an abscess, so warn the casualty that the procedure may cause significant pain.
☐ Wear sterile gloves and prepare a sterile field (*see pp.176–77*).
☐ Clean the area and infiltrate around the abscess with local anaesthetic (10ml 1% lidocaine). This will partly dull pain. Alternatively, use cold (cryogesic) spray to freeze the skin.
☐ Use a scalpel to incise firmly over the abscess into the cavity and let the pus out (be prepared with a gauze swab). Incise along the natural skin folds to minimize the scar.

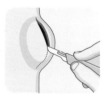

Incise firmly over the abscess.

☐ "Sweep" the abscess cavity, breaking down any walled-off areas with the handle of the scalpel or the end of a pair of forceps, to make sure all the pus is drained. This may be painful, but be firm.
☐ Prepare a long strip of gauze soaked in iodine.
☐ Pack the gauze into the abscess cavity until it is reasonably firm, leaving a tail of gauze hanging out.
☐ Apply a sterile dressing, and inspect the wound daily.
☐ Remove the gauze strip on the third day. If the wound looks clean and is not leaking pus, apply a sterile dressing. If it becomes infected again, clean the cavity and repack.

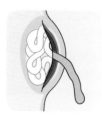

Fill the cavity with gauze soaked in iodine.

☐ Give oral antibiotics (amoxicillin + clavulanic acid).

Deep-seated or sensitive abscesses

Incision and drainage of deep abscesses or abscesses in sensitive areas may not be safe to do on the boat. Start oral antibiotics (amoxicillin + clavulanic acid) and seek medical advice. If the casualty becomes unwell with a temperature, consider changing to IV antibiotics, and arrange urgent evacuation.

LOCAL ANAESTHESIA: NERVE BLOCKS AND INFILTRATION

Local anaesthetic (LA) is very useful in managing pain during procedures such as suturing and reducing fractures.

Lidocaine is the anaesthetic agent used most often in medical kits. It is available as 1% and 2% strengths (*see* below for safe volumes to inject). Lidocaine may be mixed with adrenaline, enabling a larger dose, but only under direct medical guidance. Topical anaesthetics such as eyedrops and gels are also useful.

Indications for local anaesthesia
□ Cleaning, suturing, stapling wounds
□ Incising abscesses
□ Lower limb fracture (nerve block)
□ Damaged finger/toe (nerve block)
Cautions
□ Allergy □ Toxicity □ Pain on injection

Safe dose of local anaesthetics

All LAs are potentially toxic if too much is given too quickly. Lidocaine has a maximum safe dose.

For a 70kg crew: 20ml 1% lidocaine   or   10ml 2% lidocaine

Give proportionally more for a larger crew and less for a smaller crew.

Toxicity
Toxicity may be caused either by an excess dose or because the dose was injected directly into a blood vessel.

Initial Signs	Late Signs
□ Tingling around the mouth	□ Low blood pressure
□ Blurred vision	□ Seizures/coma
□ Slurred speech	□ Cardiac arrest

Treatment of toxicity
□ Stop giving the local anaesthetic if the casualty starts to become symptomatic.
□ For seizures, consider giving diazepam 10mg intravenously (*see* pp.172–74).
□ Treat cardiac arrest – *see* pp.48–49. Call for medical advice immediately.

Infiltration of local anaesthetic around a wound
Reducing the pain of injection
Warm the local anaesthetic to body temperature before injecting. When infiltrating around a wound, try to inject into an area already anaesthetized by a previous injection. You may wish to spray the skin first with cold (cryogesic) spray or cool it with ice.

Technique

The aim is to leave a ring of LA around the wound or site.

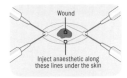

Inject anaesthetic at intervals around the wound.

□ Insert an IV cannula prior to procedure if possible, in case a bad reaction to the LA occurs.

□ Set up sterile field (see pp.176–77) and use sterile gloves.

□ Draw up the required amount of lidocaine and check it with someone else.

□ Insert the needle - usually a 23g (blue) or 25g (orange) - about 5mm under the skin, and run it in up to the hub. Pull back on the plunger at the same time to check that the needle doesn't enter a blood vessel (blood will appear if it does).

□ Start injecting and slowly pull the needle back, leaving a trail of anaesthetic.

□ Continue, using the pattern in the diagram, until the wound is encircled with LA.

□ Leave for 10 minutes and test for sensation and pain before you start.

Femoral nerve block

Seek medical advice before performing a femoral nerve block.

Indications

□ Fractured femur   □ Knee trauma   □ Lower limb fractures

Technique

□ Prepare as you would for infiltration of LA; use a 21g (green) or 23g (blue) needle.

□ Find the pulse in the groin (see diagram), which should be in the diagonal skin crease at the top of the leg; mark a point 1cm lateral to the pulse, towards the outer side of the thigh.

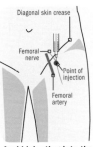

□ Insert the needle at 90° to the skin, to a depth of 30-50mm. Pull back on the plunger as you go.

□ You should feel "pops" as the needle pierces two fibrous layers

□ Make sure the needle isn't in a blood vessel and slowly inject 10-15ml 1% lidocaine.

□ If the casualty complains of an increase in pain, stop injecting, pull the needle back 5mm, and try again.

Avoid injecting into the femoral artery.

Finger and toe nerve block

The technique is similar for fingers and toes: NEVER mix adrenaline with lidocaine when anaesthetizing these areas.

Indications

This type of block is appropriate for any wound or dislocation of the finger or toe.

Technique

□ Prepare as for infiltration of LA; use a 25g (orange) needle.

□ Insert the needle on one side of the base of the finger or toe, almost through to the other side.

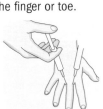

□ Pull back on the plunger to make sure the needle is not in a blood vessel.

□ Inject 2-3ml 1% lidocaine as you withdraw the needle.

Inject on both sides of the finger or toe.

□ Repeat on the other side.

□ Leave for about 10 minutes and test sensation.

□ Inject more anaesthetic under the skin, on top of and underneath the digit, if needed.

INSERTION OF TUBES AND CATHETERS

Insertion of a nasogastric (NG) tube

Indications
- Persistent vomiting
- Loss of consciousness (to deflate stomach, to reduce vomiting risk)
- Distended or rigid abdomen
- Inability to swallow (for hydration and feeding)

When NOT to insert an NG tube
- Severe facial injuries
- Suspected basal skull fracture
- When a casualty is taking blood thinning drugs, such as warfarin, to reduce clotting.

Seek medical advice before inserting an NG tube in any casualty, particularly a semi- or unconscious patient – they may vomit and then the vomit may enter the lungs.

How to insert an NG tube
- Set up for a procedure (see pp.176–77). The area does not need to be sterile, but should be clean. Use gloves.
- When you begin, the casualty should be sitting upright, if conscious, with a cup of water.
- Lubricate the nasogastric tube with petroleum jelly, cooking oil, or something similar.
- Introduce the tube to the nostril, directing it straight back, not upwards.
- As the tube passes into the nose, ask the crew to start taking frequent sips of water.
- Continue to feed the tube in through the nose. You should start to feel the tube being pulled in by the swallowing.
- If the crew gags, which is quite likely, encourage them to continue sipping.
- Aim to insert 50–60cm of tube in the average-sized male casualty. Distance measurements are marked on the tube.
- Continued coughing indicates that the tube has entered the lungs. Pull it back and try again.
- To make sure the tube is in the right place, suck some fluid from it. This fluid should look greenish/yellow. Test the acidity with urine dipsticks – the acid level (pH) should be LESS than 6 in most cases. If there is any doubt, do not put anything down the tube, and seek medical advice.
- Secure the tube firmly to the end of the nose with tape, then to the side of the face, to make sure it stays in position.
- Either attach a bag to the tube (such as a plastic bag or urine drainage bag) or, if you are feeding through the tube, put a stopper in afterwards to prevent leakage.

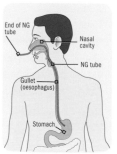

An NG tube will usually extend 45–50cms.

Insertion of a urinary catheter

Indications

- The casualty is conscious but can't pass urine despite full bladder
- The casualty is unconscious

When NOT to insert a urinary catheter

- In pelvic trauma, with blood from the penis or vagina – seek medical advice.

How to insert a urinary catheter into a male

- Set up a sterile field (see pp.176–77); use sterile gloves.
- Position the casualty on his back and put a bowl between his legs – sedation may be useful (diazepam 5mg orally).
- Gently retract the foreskin and use skin-sterilizing fluid to clean the end of the penis.
- Slowly insert local anaesthetic (lidocaine) gel into the urethra and leave it to work for 5 minutes.
- Open the catheter packet, and look at the injection port. The instructions should say how much water to inject into the balloon, which stops the catheter falling out. Fill a syringe with the correct amount (usually 5–10ml).
- Hold up the penis, pulling it gently to gain a little tension, and insert the catheter into the urethra. Feed the catheter in up to the hub. Urine should flow out into the bowl.
- Inject water into the balloon. If painful, check the catheter is all the way in and try injecting again.
- Connect the catheter to the drainage bag.
- Make sure the foreskin is put back into its normal position.
- Start antibiotics (such as ciprofloxacin) before evacuation.

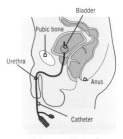

Urinary catheter in a male – side view

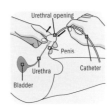

Urinary catheter in a male – insertion

How to insert a urinary catheter into a female

The procedure is essentially the same as for a male, except for the following:

- Ask a female to insert the catheter if the casualty would prefer it.
- Position the casualty with her legs apart.
- Spread the entrance to the vagina with two fingers, and clean with sterile fluid.
- Use local anaesthetic gel as outlined above.
- The entrance to the urethra is just above the entrance to the vagina (see diagram).

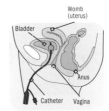

Urinary catheter in a female – side view

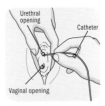

Urinary catheter in a female – insertion

Problems

The main problem is if the catheter will not pass into the bladder. There are many possible reasons this may occur. If the bladder is full and painful, a suprapubic aspiration of urine may be necessary (see p.188).

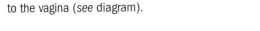

Suprapubic aspiration of urine

Indication

Use suprapubic aspiration in acute retention of urine if a normal catheter is contraindicated, for example in pelvic trauma, if there is blood from the penis or vagina.

How to aspirate urine

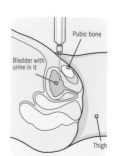

- □ Set up a sterile field (see pp.176–77), and use sterile gloves.
- □ Have the casualty lying facing upwards, and give sedation if necessary for calming (diazepam 5mg orally). Put a bowl between the legs.
- □ Feel for the pubic bone (just above the base of the penis, or at the top of the vagina). The distended and painful bladder should be palpable above this point. If not, reconsider the course of action.
- □ Clean the area and infiltrate with 5ml 1% lidocaine.
- □ Use a 21-gauge (green) needle with at least a 20ml syringe (preferably 50ml). Use a cannula if there is one available.

Insert the needle into the bladder above the pubic bone

- □ Insert the needle 2cm above the pubic bone in the midline, directing downwards (see diagram); pull back on the syringe.
- □ Urine should appear in the syringe. If it doesn't, reassess your technique. After 3 attempts, stop and seek medical advice.
- □ Once urine appears in the syringe, fill the syringe, disconnect, and squeeze the urine into the bowel. Reconnect, and repeat the process until no more urine comes out. The crew should feel relieved and be in less pain.
- □ Remove the needle and apply a sterile dressing to the site.
- □ Start antibiotics (ciprofloxacin).
- □ If urine accumulates again (as it will) and the crew member still can't urinate, you may need to either insert a catheter, or repeat this procedure.

How to insert a rectal tube

Indication

The casualty needs rehydration, but oral/nasogastric/IV routes are not available.

How to insert a rectal tube

- □ Explain what you are going to do and reassure the casualty.
- □ Position the casualty lying on the left side – right leg drawn up and left leg straight down – lying on a towel placed over a plastic sheet (the procedure can be messy).
- □ Insert a well-lubricated urinary catheter gently through the anus. Feed it in 15cm.
- □ Tape the catheter to the leg.
- □ Connect a funnel (or clean plastic bottle with the bottom cut-off) to the catheter, and slowly pour in approximately 100–150ml of fluid (for type of fluid, see p.171).
- □ The casualty may wish to defecate, but persuade them not to at this point. When the casualty does pass stool, it will increase the capacity of the rectum for fluid.
- □ Run in about 50–100ml of fluid every hour as tolerated. The rectum and colon can absorb about a maximum of 1.5L per day.

SPLINTS, CASTS, AND SLINGS

The boat's medical kit may contain a variety of splints for immobilization following an injury. There may also be plenty of material around the boat for making effective improvised splints.

SPLINTS
General rules

- The joints above and below the fracture site should be immobilized by the splint.
- Pressure points should be well padded.
- Always check the circulation before and after applying a splint.
- Remove all jewellery before applying the splint (the extremities will swell).
- Elevate the limb as far as possible after splinting.
- Periodically check perfusion and pressure points.

Malleable splint

A malleable splint is an effective, foam-covered device that can be moulded, trimmed to size, and combined with other splints. When trimming, peel back the foam and trim the aluminium underneath, and cover the end with the foam. Folding the splint into various shapes increases rigidity (see diagram).

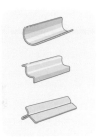

Malleable splints can be customized.

Traction splint

Traction splints are very useful for reducing and stabilizing femoral, hip, and lower leg fractures, particularly for transport. The more sophisticated splints have a gauge enabling you to measure the amount of traction force. Traction splints can be either unilateral or bilateral, the latter being more stable. When fitting a traction splint, it is vital to refer to the product instructions to avoid further damaging the leg.

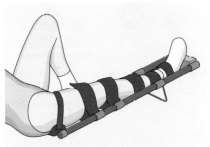

A traction splint will help to reduce a fracture, as well as immobilizing the leg or hip.

Inflatable splint

Inflatable splints are compact to carry and easier to use than vacuum splints. However, prolonged use is complicated by pressure sores and swelling of the extremities.

Vacuum splint

A vacuum splint is a polymer bag containing polystyrene beads in multiple compartments. There are different sizes of splints for upper limb, lower limb, and whole-body immobilization. The splint is placed around the site, and air is then sucked out with a special pump. The splint becomes relatively rigid but comfortable, moulded to the limb or body. Vacuum splints can be left in place for up to 24 hours.

Box splints

A lower limb or ankle fracture may be stabilized in a box splint, after initial treatment. A box-type splint can easily be improvised, following this basic design.

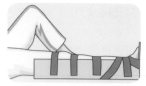

Improvised splints

Foam sleeping mattress A foam mattress can make an effective and comfortable splint if rolled up and strapped around the limb or pelvis.

Inflatable sleeping mattress Use inflatable mattresses as you would foam, except that once these are strapped on, you can inflate them to add support. Check pressure points.

Storm boards These can be used as spinal boards (covered with a camping mattress), or cut down for plain wooden arm and leg splints. Using straps or ropes, they can be fastened to the leg and used as temporary traction splints (see below).

Temporary traction splint The main requirement for a traction splint is a rigid pole or board, longer than the leg. Fasten the top firmly around the top of the thigh, with a broad strap and padding, and fasten a strap around the ankle, paying attention to pressure and perfusion. You may leave the sea boot on (cut down if necessary) to cushion the ankle and foot. Two loops of strap or rope make an effective arrangement (see diagram). Apply tension by fastening the ankle strap to the rigid splint, using a pulley system, and securing it (see diagram). Gradually increasing the tension will reduce the fracture, overcoming the thigh muscles, which may have gone into spasm.

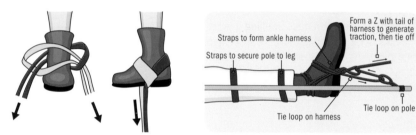

If you improvise a traction splint, make sure the straps are positioned correctly.

CASTS

Casts are made from synthetic-resin casting material, which is soaked in warm water and then applied to the limb before becoming rigid.

General rules for casts

☐ A cast will help to support a fracture if evacuation will be delayed by days.

☐ Before applying a cast, reduce fracture/dislocation, and check peripheral circulation.

☐ Do not apply the cast directly against the skin – use an under-bandage, but not tight.

☐ Do not apply the cast very tightly, just firmly. Mould it to fit before it becomes rigid.

☐ Check the circulation after applying the cast, and regularly after that.

☐ Elevate the limb as far as possible, to reduce swelling.

☐ If the peripheral circulation worsens (it may if swelling continues inside the cast), use a pair of tough-cut scissors or wire cutters to slice open one side of the cast. If circulation doesn't improve, cut the other side open as well. Monitor circulation.

SLINGS

Slings are used in addition to splints and casts to support the arm after fractures or dislocations. Your medical kit may contain a triangular bandage, which is ideal for making slings, but any cloth can be used. Slings may also reduce swelling and can help to reduce fractures gradually. The diagram (right) shows the sequence for making a broad arm sling.

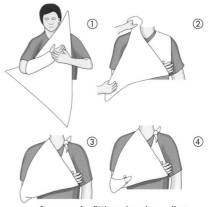

Sequence for fitting a broad arm sling

Temporary sling

A temporary sling can be made by pinning the bottom of the shirt or the shirt sleeve to the fabric on the upper chest, with the arm inside.

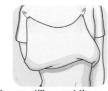

You can still support the arm if there is no material available for making a sling.

High arm sling

This sling is used to reduce swelling in wrist or hand fractures. Wrap the sling as you would a typical broad arm sling (above), except start with the triangular bandage on the outside of the arm, rather than the inside.

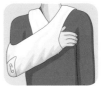

A high arm sling protects and elevates the wrist and hand.

Broad arm sling

Broad arm slings may be used for fractures and dislocations of the shoulder, clavicle, and upper and lower arms, including the elbow. A bandage or tape, as shown in the Collar and Cuff diagram (below right), can be wrapped around the upper body, under the good arm, to reduce involuntary movement of the broken arm and sling.

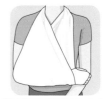

Broad arm slings are used for support in a range of fractures and dislocations.

Collar and cuff sling

A collar and cuff sling is used for a fracture of the humerus (upper arm). The fracture may reduce slowly with the gentle weight of the lower arm. Bandaging around the entire upper body, including the sling, will provide extra support.

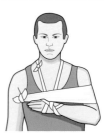

A collar and cuff sling can help to reduce fractures.

REDUCING FRACTURES AND DISLOCATIONS

The aim in reducing all fractures and dislocations is to return the bones to their normal position. This should reduce pain, increase mobility, reduce the threat to the blood and nerve supply, and reduce the risk of infection in open fractures.

Overall treatment involves prompt reduction, cleaning and dressing of wounds (especially those involving fractured bones – for more information on fractures, *see* pp.98–103), and applying splints, casts, and traction as required (see p.189).

Fractures may be:

Displaced The ends of the bones are put out of place to either side.
Angulated The ends of the bone are at an angle to each other.
Rotated The ends are rotated in opposite directions. This type of fracture can occur when sheets or ropes become wrapped around a limb and then come under load.

Displaced fracture   Angulated fracture   Rotated fracture

General technique for reducing a fracture or dislocation

Aim to begin as soon as possible and before the muscles go in to spasm, which will tend to shorten the limb, making successful reduction more difficult.

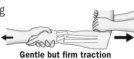

Gentle but firm traction for 5–10 minutes

- Find a stable position, and take usual precautions for setting up a procedure (*see* pp.176–77).
- The casualty has to be relaxed and have plenty of analgesia. The procedure will be very painful:
  - sedation: diazepam 5–10mg orally
  - analgesia: morphine 5mg IM (repeat if necessary) or tramadol 100mg IV or methoxyflurane inhaler (one only)

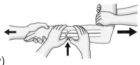

Press bones into normal position.

- Use gentle but firm traction. Reducing the fracture may take 10–30 minutes, so be patient and persist. Give more analgesia if required.
- Bones may return to the usual position with traction only
- If they do not, try easing the fractured ends back together using direct pressure (see diagram).
- If any of these manoeuvres increase the pain significantly, reconsider what you are doing. Assess the blood and nerve supply (check capillary refill time, *see* p.167; and test sensation). You may need to splint or support the limb as it is.
- Before releasing traction, apply a splint to the limb (*see* pp.188–89 & pp.193–195).
- Check blood and nerve supply after reducing a fracture or dislocation, and repeat check at frequent intervals until the casualty is evacuated.

Specific fractures and dislocations

Dislocated shoulder
Try either of the methods below (designed for frontal dislocations), but stop if bone grating (crepitus) occurs, and support the arm in a sling.

Method 1
□ Lie the casualty facing upwards, grasp the dislocated arm around the wrist, and gently, slowly lift it to a vertical position.
□ When the arm is vertical, apply traction.
□ Maintaining vertical traction, rotate the arm externally.
□ If you experience difficulty, it may assist reduction if you locate the head of the humerus, in the armpit, and gently push it in towards the socket, maintaining traction with the other hand.

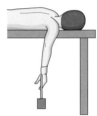

Relocating shoulder:
method 1

Method 2
□ Lie casualty face down on the galley table or on a bunk with the dislocated arm on the outside; pad under the shoulder.
□ Attach a 2–4kg weight to the arm, in the position shown in the diagram. The weight you apply will depend on the size and musculature of the casualty.
□ Relaxation, traction, and reduction of the arm may take longer than 30 minutes.
□ After relocation, use a broad arm sling to support the arm.

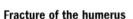
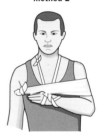

Relocating shoulder:
method 2

Fracture of the humerus
Only attempt reduction of upper-arm fractures if blood and nerve supply are compromised. If you do, use the general technique described above. Otherwise, treat with a collar and cuff splint (wrap a bandage around the body and the sling for extra support if conditions are rough). In this position the fracture may reduce by itself. For further support, apply a back slab to the upper arm.

Collar and cuff splint

Elbow fractures and dislocations
In elbow injuries, the lower arm is nearly always pushed backwards through the elbow joint. The bone may be only dislocated or may be fractured as well. The elbow may look slightly bent, but should straighten after reduction.
□ Apply traction along the line of the arm, with an assistant holding the upper arm (see illustration, left).
□ As the muscles relax, try bending the arm straight gently.

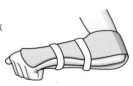

Elbow splint

□ A "clunk" may indicate that the elbow has relocated.
□ Support the elbow with a splint (see diagram) and a broad arm sling.
□ Check blood and nerve supply, as elbow injuries carry a significant risk of damage to blood vessels and nerves.

Forearm and wrist fractures

Use the general technique for reduction described on page 192 and immobilize with a splint that extends around the elbow and down to the hand (see elbow splint diagram, previous page). Curl the hand and fingers over something soft (such as rolled-up gauze). If evacuation will take longer than a few days, the splint can be replaced with a back slab when time and conditions allow. This should run from above elbow (held at 90°) to the hand (*see* diagram, right). Support the arm with a broad arm sling. NEVER apply a full cast to a new fracture – only a back slab. The arm will swell, and pressure increase inside a full cast, cutting off blood supply.

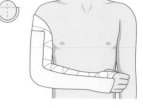

Forearm back slab

Finger and toe fractures and dislocations

Perform reduction quickly after the injury, before full sensation returns. If there is a delay, a ring block may be needed to ease the pain and allow reduction (*see* p.185).

□ Pull the distal part of the finger (*see* diagram). There may be a pop when it relocates. The joint may require some pushing to get it back in line.

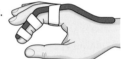

Relocating a finger

□ Tape to an adjoining finger with a pad of gauze in-between. If an open wound prevents buddy splinting, use the arrangement in the diagram – a piece of flexible splint moulded along the back of the hand.

Flexible finger splint

□ Keep the digit immobilized for a week or so if you think the injury was a dislocation: keep fractures immobilized for several weeks.

Hip dislocation

The hip normally dislocates backwards and leaves the leg rotated towards the midline. This may happen in a casualty with a hip replacement, and it is the replacement parts that dislocate. Relocation requires very firm traction and will cause considerable pain: use diazepam and morphine or tramadol – *see* General technique, p.192.

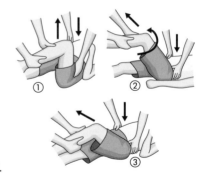

Relocating the hip

□ Position the casualty lying facing upwards.
□ Slowly bend the hip to 90° (**1**). This will hurt.
□ Keep casualty's lower leg between your legs.
□ Pull up on the lower leg behind the knee, while an assistant presses down on the casualty's pelvis, to keep it from rising off the floor (**2**).
□ As the hip relocates over time, rotate the thigh inwards (**3**) then carefully lie the leg down and strap it to the other leg, using padding in-between.
□ If there is a traction splint available, gentle traction may help to keep the hip in place.
□ Do not make more than three attempts. Check blood and nerve supply each time.

Pelvic fracture

A dedicated pelvic splint or binder may be included in the medical kit, or can be fashioned from equipment on-board. The binder may be in place for a prolonged period, so should be of soft material. The band should be centred on the "hip bones" (greater trochanters), and tightened so that a finger can still be inserted between it and the skin. It should stay in place until the casualty is evacuated.

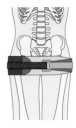

Pelvic splint

Femoral fracture

A traction splint is ideal for this major fracture of the thigh bone. There are many types of traction splints with different methods of application (e.g. on p.190), but in general you can follow these steps. Other injuries may be present, so carry out an assessment.

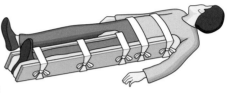

Improvised immobilization splint

- Provide as much analgesia as necessary, including femoral nerve block (*see* p.185).
- Try fitting the traction splint to the uninjured leg, to take measurements, before moving the injured side.
- Use only as much traction as is necessary to reduce the deformity.
- Check blood and nerve supply before and after applying the splint.

If a traction splint is not available, make a simple immobilization splint by strapping storm boards, or something similar, down each side of the leg, from the armpit to below the feet (*see* illustration, above). Strap the legs together for extra support. Use plenty of padding between the splints and the leg and between the knees and ankles.

Lower leg fracture

Lower leg fractures are reduced by a similar method to fractured forearms. It is possible to use a traction splint for controlled, gentle traction to reduce deformity. A box splint (*see* p.190) will adequately immobilize the leg, as will a malleable splint in a U shape (see diagram). It is very important to elevate the leg to reduce swelling, which may be severe. *Do not apply a cast encircling the leg*, as the swelling may increase the pressure and cut off the circulation.

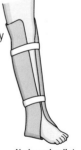

Ankle fracture and dislocation

U-shaped splint

The injury may be a combined fracture and dislocation, and hard to diagnose on a boat. Blood and nerve supply may be compromised. Reducing the fracture and/or dislocation requires reasonable force and will be painful – use adequate analgesia.

- Apply traction to the foot, with an assistant holding the leg.
- Aim to get the ankle in line with the lower leg, with the foot in the normal position at 90° to the lower leg.
- Apply a U-shaped splint (see diagram above), keeping the foot at 90°.
- Check blood and nerve supply, readjusting the splint if the limb is too restricted.

Appendices

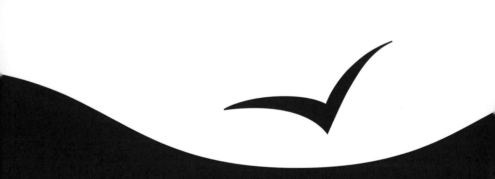

- Medical Screening Questionnaire
- Vital Signs Monitoring Chart
- Medical Reporting Chart
- Immunizations Guide
- Medical Kit List
- Guide to Commonly Used Drugs
- Pain Relief Ladder
- Antibiotics Guide
- Helicopter Evacuation
- Life Raft Evacuation Procedure
- Man Overboard
- Dealing with a Death On-board

MEDICAL SCREENING QUESTIONNAIRE

CONFIDENTIAL – DO NOT DISCLOSE UNLESS IN AN EMERGENCY

Name: _____

Date of birth/age: _____

Occupation: _____

Address: _____

Contact number: _____

Email: _____

Next of kin: _____

□ Please record details of any medical conditions from which you suffer.

_____

_____

Specifically, have you ever suffered from:
- High blood pressure .... Yes ☐ No ☐
- Heart attacks (myocardial infarctions/coronaries) .... Yes ☐ No ☐
- Angina .... Yes ☐ No ☐
- Strokes (cerebral vascular accidents) .... Yes ☐ No ☐
- Jaundice .... Yes ☐ No ☐
- Tuberculosis .... Yes ☐ No ☐
- Rheumatic fever .... Yes ☐ No ☐
- Diabetes .... Yes ☐ No ☐
- Epilepsy .... Yes ☐ No ☐
- Asthma .... Yes ☐ No ☐
- Depression .... Yes ☐ No ☐
- Blood infections, such as hepatitis A, B, or C, or human immunodeficiency virus (HIV) .... Yes ☐ No ☐
- Chronic back pain .... Yes ☐ No ☐
- Kidney stones .... Yes ☐ No ☐
- Cartilage/ligament injuries .... Yes ☐ No ☐
- Musculoskeletal injuries .... Yes ☐ No ☐
- Gynaecological problems .... Yes ☐ No ☐
- Organ transplants, chemotherapy, or steroids .... Yes ☐ No ☐

□ **If yes to any of the above, please record details:**

_____

_____

□ Are there any inherited medical conditions in your family? Please include details:

_____

_____

□ Have you had any operations? Please include details and dates:

_____

_____

_____

□ Please record any medications that you take or have taken in the past, either regularly or occasionally (please include herbal or alternative medicines):

_____

_____

□ Are you allergic to anything? Please include details of circumstances and reactions:

_____

_____

□ Do you smoke or drink alcohol? Please include quantities:

_____

_____

□ Do you suffer from indigestion or heartburn? .... Yes ☐ No ☐

□ Please record details of any dental work that you may have undergone, together with an assessment of the present state of your teeth:

_____

_____

□ Do you have any physical disabilities? Please include details:

_____

_____

□ Do you suffer from seasickness?

_____

_____

Yes☐ No☐
- If yes, on a scale of 1–10 (10 is worst),
  how sick are you?
  1☐ 2☐ 3☐ 4☐ 5☐ 6☐ 7☐ 8☐ 9☐ 10☐

- What preventative measures do you
  normally take?

  _____

  _____

□ Are you colour blind?...........Yes☐ No☐
- If yes, which colours are involved?

_____

_____

_____

□ Please detail all immunizations you have
  had, together with dates:

  _____

  _____

  _____

□ What is your blood group? _____
□ What is your height? _____
□ What is your weight? _____
□ For insurance purposes, have you received
  medical advice or treatment during the
  previous 12 months relating to any illness,
  disability or condition whatsoever?
                              Yes☐ No☐

If yes, please detail:

  _____

  _____

  _____

**I confirm that I have answered the above questionnaire truthfully and to the best of
my ability.**

Signed and dated_____

FROM YOUR USUAL FAMILY DOCTOR

Practice's name, address, and contact number:

_____

_____

_____

Please state how long you have been the above person's family doctor: _____

I declare that to the best of my knowledge and belief that the statements and particulars
detailed in this questionnaire are true and complete.

Signed _____

_____

Date _____

VITAL SIGNS MONITORING CHART

Crew name: _____ Boat: _____

Temperature °C (Site)			00:00	1:00	2:00	3:00	4:00	5:00	6:00	7:00	8:00	9:00	
		40											
		39											
		38											
		37											
		36											
		35											
		34											
Pulse and Blood Pressure (mmHg)		190											
		180											
		170											
		160											
		150											
		140											
		130											
		120											
		110											
		100											
		90											
		80											
		70											
		60											
		50											
		40											
		30											
Time			00:00	1:00	2:00	3:00	4:00	5:00	6:00	7:00	8:00	9:00	
Glasgow Coma Score	Eyes	4											
		3											
		2											
		1											
	Verbal	5											
		4											
		3											
		2											
		1											
	Motor	6											
		5											
		4											
		3											
		2											
		1											
	TOTAL												
Oxygen Saturation %													
Respiratory Rate BPM													
Urine Output mls													

Date: _____   **Location:** _____

10:00	11:00	12:00	13:00	14:00	15:00	16:00	17:00	18:00	19:00	20:00	21:00	22:00	23:00

MEDICAL REPORTING CHART

A detailed medical report should accompany the casualty who is being evacuated, whether to another ship, directly on to the quayside, or via a helicopter. The purpose of the report is to inform the doctors on shore about exactly what happened to the casualty, what treatment they have received, and how they have progressed. It should give an indication as to possible diagnosis and what treatments are required next.

A structured report is much easier to understand than a long rambling letter – bear in mind that it may be read by doctors whose first language is not your own. A written report is also easier to understand than a verbal report and is an enduring record of what happened on the boat. You should keep a copy.

The information that should be covered includes:
- Patient's name, date of birth, home address and next of kin, together with contact details
- The main reason (illness or trauma) why the casualty is being evacuated, including circumstances and timing of events
- The current vital signs observations, together with any observation charts already completed
- The treatments already given and the casualty's responses, including any information from doctors in previous ports
- All other details about the patient, including previous medical history, normal medications, and allergies
- Details of the captain of the boat and the crew member who was responsible for treating the casualty. These details may be important if the doctors on shore require further information.

If you are unsure whether to include certain information, put it in rather than leave it out. The medical report must be confidential, and it should be used only for the purpose of treating the casualty. It should not be passed to any third party without the express consent of the casualty.

Medical Report—Confidential	Name:
Ship's name:	DoB:
Position of evacuation:	Date: ﹐
MAIN COMPLAINT	Date of onset or incident:

History:

Examination:

Vital signs: Pulse Respiratory rate GCS
Blood presssure Temperature Urine

Treatment:

Past medical history:

High blood pressure/Angina/Heart attacks/Jaundice/TB/Rheumatic fever/Diabetes/Epilepsy/Asthma

Normal medications:

Allergies:

Next of kin:

Copies: Ship's copy Shore copy Signature:

Print name:

IMMUNIZATIONS GUIDE

□ The geographical extent of various diseases changes with time – consult a local health agency for current recommendations.

□ Some vaccines cannot be given to the very young or to people with particular medical problems: Seek medical advice.

Disease	Geographical Area	Immunization Schedule	Period	Notes
Cholera	Africa, South America, S. & S.E. Asia, Middle East, India, Caribbean	A course of 2 oral doses 1-6 weeks apart, finishing 1 week before travel	2 years	A booster dose up to 2 years after the initial course prolongs protection
Hepatitis A	India, Africa, Central and South America, East Asia, Middle East	1 injection 2 weeks before travel	About 1 year	A second injection 6-12 months after the first gives protection for up to 20 years
Japanese encephalitis	Southeast and East Asia, northeast Australia, Pacific Islands	A course of 2 injections over 30 days, finishing 1 month before travel	1-2 years	A shorter course is available but gives a shorter period of lower level protection
Meningococcal disease (A, C, Y, W135 types)	Worldwide (particularly Sub-Saharan Africa, Middle East, India)	1 quadrivalent injection 2-3 weeks before travel	5 years or more	A quadrivalent vaccine protects against A, C, Y, W135 types)
Poliomyelitis	Sub-Saharan Africa, Indian subcontinent	1 booster dose if vaccinated more than 10 years ago, or 1 booster dose for high-risk areas	10 years	Will require 3 doses if never previously vaccinated
Tetanus	Worldwide	1 booster dose if vaccinated more than 10 years previously	10 years	Will require up to 3 doses if never previously vaccinated
Tick-borne encephalitis	Forested areas of central, western, and eastern Europe, Russia, China, Japan	A course of three injections over 5-12 months	Up to 3 years	A shorter course is available but gives a shorter period of lower level protection
Typhoid	Asia, Africa, India, Central and South America, Middle East, Europe	1 injection/3 oral capsules 30 days before travel	3 years	Not 100% effective, so take care with food/water hygiene
Yellow fever	Sub-Saharan Africa, South America	1 injection /booster 10 days before travel	10 years	Some countries require a certificate of vaccination on entry

MEDICAL KIT LIST

On the following pages, lists are supplied for three medical kits: the grab bag kit, the inside helicopter range (IHR) kit, and the outside helicopter range (OHR) kit. The grab bag, as the name implies, is the medical kit you should grab if abandoning the boat and taking to the life raft. At other times, the grab bag should be considered an integral part of both the IHR and OHR kits: while you are on board, you always need access to either the grab bag plus the IHR kit or the grab bag plus the OHR kit.

The grab bag includes basic equipment for treatment of injuries that may have been sustained during the disaster that cause the abandonment. It also includes medications such as antiseasickness treatments and painkillers, which will be essential on a life raft.

The IHR kit is designed for boats with a crew of up to 10 people, operating within 240–320 km (150–200 miles) of a port with good medical facilities, or within helicopter range. The OHR kit is designed for boats with a crew of up to 10 people, operating outside the range of helicopters (beyond approximately 240–320 km).

These lists are a guide to what should be included in boat medical kits, operating under the conditions described above. They are based upon both guidelines issued by various statutory authorities (for local authorities, see p.219) and on personal experience of treating trauma and illnesses on vessels at sea. The lists also take account of what is practicable to store on smaller boats.

Every expedition is different, as is every crew. The medical kit should be examined critically prior to leaving port, to make sure it contains specific treatments the crew members might require (in the light of their medical history), and also to cover special risks that may be incurred by the expedition route, such as whether it will pass through malarial regions or polar regions. There are additional items not included in the IHR and OHR kit lists that may be considered worthy of inclusion, depending on the logistics of the expedition.

Oxygen therapy	IV fluid	Defibrillator
□ Oxygen cylinder or concentrator □ Pressure regulator □ Tubing □ Face masks of differing sizes	□ IV cannulas □ Cannula dressings □ Giving sets □ IV fluid (5–10L of Ringer's/ normal saline)	□ Marine defibrillator □ Pads □ Monitoring electrodes □ Service schedule

Using defibrillators, oxygen therapy, and IV fluid requires special training, medical advice at the time of use, and attention to maintaining the skills necessary to use this equipment safely.

ITEM

FIRST AID

Item	GRAB BAG/QTY	IHR KIT/QTY	OHR KIT/QTY
Assorted waterproof plasters, box	1	1	1
Paracetamol 500mg	100	100	100
Ibuprofen 400mg	84	84	84
Diclofenac supps 100mg	10		10
Aspirin 300mg			32
Tramadol 50mg		100	100
Adhesive skin tape 12mmx100mm, 6 pack	6	6	6
Adhesive elastic bandage 7.5cmx4.5m, roll		4	4
Adhesive elastic strapping 2.5cmx4.5m, roll		2	2
Tough cut scissors, pair	1	1	1
Head torch	1	1	1
Disposable scalpel	10	5	10
Trauma tourniquet		1	1

EMERGENCY/ALLERGY

Item	GRAB BAG/QTY	IHR KIT/QTY	OHR KIT/QTY
Atropine 600mcg inj		10	10
Adrenaline (epinephrine) 1:1000 inj	4	10	10
Prednisolone 5mg	28	28	28
Hydrocortisone 100mg inj		5	5
Chlorphenamine 10mg inj		2	2
Salbutamol 100mcg inh	1	1	1
Beclometasone 100mcg inh	1	1	1
Loratadine 10mg	30	30	60
Cetirizine 10mg		30	60
Oxytocin + ergometrine 5iu inj		5	5
Glyceryltrinitrate spray 400mcg	1	1	1
Glyceryltrinitrate patch 5mg		30	30
Furosemide 40mg		28	56
Furosemide 20mg inj			10
Atenolol 50mg			28
Diazepam 10mg inj			10
Diazepam 5mg			28
Diazepam 10mg (rectal dispenser)		5	5
Chlorpromazine 25mg		28	28
Chlorpromazine 25mg inj			10
Dextrose gel 20g	1	1	1

ANALGESICS

Item	GRAB BAG/QTY	IHR KIT/QTY	OHR KIT/QTY
Lidocaine 1% 5ml amp		10	10
Lidocaine gel 6ml			2
Ethyl chloride spray		1	1
Ibuprofen gel 100g		1	2
Choline salicylate dental gel 15g		2	2
Codeine 15mg		56	56

ITEM

ANTIBIOTICS

Item	GRAB BAG/QTY	IHR KIT/QTY	OHR KIT/QTY
Amoxicillin + clavulananic acid 625mg	42	42	42
Amoxicillin + clavulananic acid 600mg inj		10	20
Water for inj 10ml		10	20
Ciprofloxacin 500mg	20	40	40
Flucloxacillin 500mg	28	28	56
Metronidazole 400mg	21	21	21
Metronidazole supp 1g			20
Doxycycline 100mg		50	50
Fusidic acid 2% ointment 30g		1	1
Ear/eye drops (antibiotic/steroid) 10ml		2	2
Ceftriaxone 1g inj			10
Tetanus vaccine (combined with diphtheria)		2	5
Mebendazole 100mg		6	6
Clotrimazole pessary 500mg (applicator)		1	1
Clotrimazole 1% cream 20g		1	1

CD DRUGS

Item	GRAB BAG/QTY	IHR KIT/QTY	OHR KIT/QTY
Morphine 10mg inj	20		
Cyclizine 50mg inj	10		
Naloxone 400mcg, 3 pack	1		
Tramadol 100mg inj	20		
Blue needles 23g and 2.5/5ml Syringes	10		

GUT/SEASICKNESS

Item	GRAB BAG/QTY	IHR KIT/QTY	OHR KIT/QTY
Cinnarizine 15mg	84	84	84
Domperidone 10mg	30	30	30
Promethazine 25mg	10	10	10
Prochlorperazine 3mg	50	50	50
Ondansetron 4mg	10	10	10
Hyoscine hydrobromide 0.3mg		60	60
Lansoprazole 15mg		56	56
Lactulose 500ml, bottle			1
Bisacodyl 5mg			60
Glycerin supps 4g		12	12
Loperamide 2mg		60	60
Rehydration salts (powder sachets)		20	40
Hyoscine butylbromide 10mg		40	40
Haemorrhoid cream/oint 25g		2	2

BURNS/EYES/SKIN/NOSE

Item	GRAB BAG/QTY	IHR KIT/QTY	OHR KIT/QTY
Chloramphenicol eye ointment 4g tube		2	4
Tetracaine minims 0.5%		20	20
Dexamethasone 0.1% 0.5ml minims		20	20

Note All drugs specified are in tablet form unless otherwise stated.

Burns/eyes/skin/nose cont.

ITEM	GRAB BAG/QTY	IHR KIT/QTY	OHR KIT/QTY
Aciclovir 5% cream 2g		1	1
Pilocarpine 0.5% 10ml		1	1
Hypromellose 1% 10ml		1	1
Fluorescein 2% 0.5ml minims		20	20
Tropicamide 1% 0.5ml minims		20	20
Normal saline sterile pods 10mls		5	10
Pseudoephedrine 60mg		24	24
Silver sulfadiazine 50g	1	1	2
Burn bag	2	2	2
Burn dressing 10x10cm		1	1
Burn dressing 20x20cm		1	1
Chlorhexidine gluconate 0.2% 300ml		1	1
Paraffin gauze dressing 10cmx10cm		10	10
Antiseptic cleansing solution 25ml		20	40
Hydrocortisone cream 1% 15g tube			1
Miconazole cream 2% 45g			1
Permethrin 1% rinse 59ml			1
Magnesium sulphate paste		1	1
Mupirocin cream 2% 15g		1	1

DRESSINGS/SPLINTS/CASTS

ITEM	GRAB BAG/QTY	IHR KIT/QTY	OHR KIT/QTY
Tubular elasticated bandage 1m size D/B/F	1	1	1
Malleable arm/hand splint	1	1	1
Sterile gauze pads 7.5cmx7.5cm, 5 pack	5	5	5
Non-adherent dressings 5cmx5cm	10	20	20
Sterile dressings	2	3	3
Microporous surgical tape 2.5mx10m			2
Crepe bandage 7.5cmx4m	1	2	1
Triangular bandage cloth	2	4	4
Semirigid neck collar	1		
Leg/thigh traction splint		1	1
Malleable finger splint		2	2
Tubular gauze finger bandage with applicator		1	1
Inflatable splints (leg and arm)		2	2

SKIN REPAIR

ITEM	GRAB BAG/QTY	IHR KIT/QTY	OHR KIT/QTY
Toothed forceps		1	1
Tweezer forceps		1	1
Artery clamps		1	1
5" sh/sh scissors		1	1
2/0 silk sutures		2	6
3/0 vicryl sutures			6
Skin adhesive		1	2

Skin repair cont.

ITEM	GRAB BAG/QTY	IHR KIT/QTY	OHR KIT/QTY
Skin stapler		2	2
Staple remover		1	1
Antiseptic surgical fluid 500ml			1
Gloves sterile, medium pair		5	5
Gloves sterile, large pair		5	5
Gloves nonsterile, large pair		15	20
Foley catheters 14G & 16G			2
Drainage bag 2L			1
Nasogastric tubes 14F (Ryles tubes)			1
Stethoscope	1		
Sphygmomanometer, handheld aneroid model	1		
Foil blankets	1	1	1
BP cuff 15x7 Velcro S Tube		1	1
Otoscope		1	1
Digital thermometer		1	1
Pregnancy testing kit, double pack			1
Urinalysis diagnostic testing strips (50s), pack		1	1
Blood glucose testing meter		1	1
Magnifying glass		1	1
Guedel airways, sizes 3 & 4		2	2
Nasopharyngeal airways, 6mm & 8mm		2	2
Resuscitator, reuseable, with reservoir		1	1
Emergency aspirator and 2 catheters		1	1
Oxygen reservoir 400L		1	1
Pocket face mask with valve		1	1
Emergency medical treatment manual		1	1
Vital signs chart		6	6
Medical report sheet		6	6

DENTAL

ITEM	GRAB BAG/QTY	IHR KIT/QTY	OHR KIT/QTY
Dental kit			1

IV FLUIDS

ITEM	GRAB BAG/QTY	IHR KIT/QTY	OHR KIT/QTY
IV fluid (Ringer's/normal saline) 1 L			6
IV giving sets			2

EQUIPMENT

ITEM	GRAB BAG/QTY	IHR KIT/QTY	OHR KIT/QTY
Cannula 16g/20g			10
Transparent cannula dressing			10
5ml syringes	5	5	5
10ml syringes	5	5	5
Green needles 21G	10	20	20
Injection swabs	10	10	10
Normal saline 10ml plastic vials			10

Abbreviations: **IHR** = Inside Helicopter Range **OHR** = Outside Helicopter Range **amp** = ampoule **inh** = inhaler **inj** = injection **supp** = suppository

GUIDE TO COMMONLY USED DRUGS

Medicine	Indication	Adult Dose	Common Side Effects
Aciclovir 5% cream	Cold sores (herpes simplex)	5 times daily for 5–10 days	Start at first sign of attack. May cause stinging, dry skin. Avoid eyes
Aciclovir 3% oint	Herpes simplex eye infections	1 application 5 times a day for at least 3 days	Local inflammation, irritation
Aciclovir (tab)	Herpes simplex viral infections	400–800mg 3–5 times a day for 5 days or more	Maintain good hydration. Abdominal pain, diarrhoea, nausea, rash, sun sensitivity
Amiodarone (IV inj)	Resuscitation (see p.31)	300mg IV once only	Only for use in resuscitation
Amoxicillin	Ear/general infections	250–1,000mg tds	Avoid in penicillin allergy. May cause stomach upset
Amoxicillin + clavulanic acid (IV inj)	Severe chest/dental/gut infections	600–1,200mg IV tds	Avoid in penicillin allergy. May cause stomach upset
Amoxicillin + clavulanic acid (tab)	Chest/dental/gut infections	375–625mg tds	Avoid in penicillin allergy. May cause stomach upset
Aspirin	Mild pain; heart attack	300–900mg qds	Avoid with indigestion, stomach ulcers, asthma
Atenolol	Antihypertensive	25–50mg od	May cause low pulse rate, low blood pressure, wheeze, fatigue, cold limbs
Azithromycin	Chest infections	500mg od for 3 days	May cause stomach upset, abdominal pain
Beclometasone	Asthma/wheeze	2 puffs bd	Few short term side effects
Bisacodyl	Constipation (stimulant)	5–10mg at night	May cause abdominal cramps, griping
Ceftriaxone (IM or IV inj)	Severe chest/gut infections	1g od IM or IV – 2g	May cause stomach upset, abdominal pain
Cetirizine	Antihistamine	10mg od	Low risk of drowsiness, urinary retention, blurred vision
Chloramphenicol 0.5% eye drops or ointment 1%	Eye infections	1 application/4 h until infection improves. Use for 48 h	Transient stinging. Avoid prolonged use
Chlorphenamine IM inj	Antihistamine, anti-allergy	10–20mg (max: 40mg in 24 h)	Drowsiness, urinary retention, blurred vision, transient low blood pressure
Chlorphenamine (tab)	Antihistamine, anti-allergy	4mg 3–6 times a day (max: 24mg in 24 h)	Drowsiness, urinary retention, blurred vision, transient low blood pressure
Chlorpromazine (IM inj)	Severe anxiety/psychosis	25–50mg IM 6–8 hourly	Drowsiness, low blood pressure, tremor, abnormal movements
Chlorpromazine (tab)	Severe anxiety/psychosis	25–100mg tds	Drowsiness, low blood pressure, tremor, abnormal movements

Note: Always refer to the specific medicine information leaflet for further information

Abbreviations:

amp = ampoule	**IV** = intravenous inj	**supp** = suppository	**od** = once a day
IM = intramucular inj	**pr** = rectal route	**SC** = subcutaneous	**qds** = 4 times a day
inj = injection	**tab** = tablet	**bd** = twice a day	**tds** = 3 times a day

Medicine	Indication	Adult Dose	Common Side Effects
Choline salicylate dental gel	Mouth sores	Apply bd or qds	Occasional worsening of irritation or infection—do not use for infections
Cinnarizne	Seasickness	15mg tds	May cause drowsiness, fatigue, blurred vision
Ciprofloxacin	Gut/urinary infections	250-500mg bd	Caution in epilepsy. May cause tendonitis
Codydramol	Moderate pain	2 tabs every 6 h (max 8 tabs in 24 h)	Not with other drugs containing paracetamol. Avoid with liver disease
Clotrimazole (pessary)	Vaginal fungal infection	500mg pessary once only	A repeat dose may be required after a week
Codeine	Moderate pain	40mg every 4-6 h	Avoid with respiratory depression, head injury
Cyclizine (IM inj)	Sickness caused by morphine	50mg IM tds	May cause drowsiness. Painful injection
Dexamethasone 0.1% eye drops	Inflammation of the eye	3-4 drops every 4-6 h	Seek medical advice before using in a 'red eye' or with signs of infection
Diazepam (IM inj)	Seizures (see p.40)	5-10mg IM, as needed	May cause drowsiness, confusion, respiratory depression
Diazepam (supp)	Seizures (see p.40)	10mg, pr	May cause drowsiness, confusion, respiratory depression
Diazepam (tab)	Seizures/anxiety/muscle spasm	5-10mg every 2 h, as needed	May cause drowsiness, confusion, respiratory depression
Diclofenac (supp)	Moderate pain	75mg bd pr	Avoid with indigestion, stomach ulcers, asthma
Diclofenac (tab)	Moderate pain	50mg tds	Avoid with indigestion, stomach ulcers, asthma
Dihydrocodeine	Moderate pain	40mg every 4-6 h	Avoid with respiratory depression, head injury
Domperidone (tab)	Seasickness	10-20mg qds	May occasionally cause stomach cramps
Doxycycline (tab)	Chest/gut/ear infections, malaria prophylaxis	100mg od	May cause stomach upset, abdominal pain, skin sun sensitivity
Epinephrine (adrenaline) (IM inj)	Resuscitation, anaphylaxis	See p.31 and p.50	Only for use in resuscitation and anaphylaxis
Erythromycin	Chest/gut/ear infections	250-500mg tds	May cause stomach upset, abdominal pain
Eye and ear drops (antibiotic/steriod)	Inflammation/infection of the outer ear or eye	2-3 drops every 6-8 h	Seek medical advice before using in a "red eye" or with signs of infection
Flucloxacillin	Skin infections	250-500mg qds	Avoid in penicillin allergy. May cause stomach upset
Flumazenil	Sleeping pill overdose		To be used only under the medical direction of a doctor
Fluorescein 2% eye drops	Staining to detect foreign bodies and eye lesions	3-4 drops once	Results in a yellow eye for several hours
Furosemide (IV inj)	Heart failure (diuretic)	20-40mg IV od	May cause low blood pressure, dizziness
Furosemide (tab)	Heart failure (diuretic)	20-40mg od	May cause low blood pressure, dizziness

Drug	Indication	Adult Dose	Common Side Effects
Fusidic acid 2% ointment (Fucidin)	Skin infections	Apply od–tds	Local irritation, itching, burning
Glyceryltrinitrate (patch)	Angina, heart attack	1–2 patches, as needed. Replace od	May cause low blood pressure, flushing, headache, fast heart rate
Glyceryltrinitrate (spray under tongue)	Angina, heart attack	1–2 sprays, as needed	May cause low blood pressure, flushes, headache, fast heart rate; use under medical direction
Hydrocortisone (IM or IV inj)	Anti-allergy	100mg IM or IV, tds, as needed	May cause indigestion, abdominal discomfort
Hydrocortisone 1% cream	Mild inflammatory skin disorders (eczema, bites)	Apply thinly od or bd	May cause worsening of infection if present. Avoid prolonged use
Hyoscine butylbromide	Antibowel spasm/colic	10–20mg qds	May cause dry mouth, blurred vision, constipation
Hyoscine hydrobromide (patch)	Seasickness	1 patch behind ear. Replace every 72 h	May cause drowsiness, blurred vision, urinary retention
Hyoscine hydrobromide (tab)	Seasickness	0.3mg bd	May cause drowsiness, blurred vision, urinary retention
Ibuprofen	Mild–moderate pain	400mg every 4–6 h	Avoid with indigestion, stomach ulcers, asthma
Lactulose	Constipation (softens stool)	15ml bd	May cause flatulance, cramps, abdominal discomfort
Lansoprazole	Indigestion, reflux	15–30mg od	May cause stomach upset, diarrhoea, constipation, headache
Lidocaine (SC inj)	Local anesthetic inj	See p.184	See p.184
Loperamide	Diarrhoea	4mg; then 2mg/each loose stool. Max 16mg in 24 h	May cause abdominal cramps, dizziness, drowsiness, bloating
Loratadine	Antihistamine	10mg od	Low risk of drowsiness, urinary retention, blurred vision
Lorazepam (IV inj)	Seizures (see p.40)	2–4mg, as needed	May cause drowsiness, confusion, respiratory depression. Use only under direction of a doctor
Mebendazole	Gut worm infections	100mg bd for 3 days	May cause abdominal pain, diarrhoea
Methoxyflurane inhaler (Penthrox®)	Moderate to severe pain associated with trauma	3–6ml by inhaler. Avoid on consecutive days	Avoid in liver or renal disease, or diabetes. Use only under direction of a doctor
Metronidazole (supp)	Gut/dental infections	1g tds pr	May cause nausea and vomiting (worse if taken with alcohol)
Metronidazole (tab)	Gut/dental infections	400mg tds	May cause nausea and vomiting (worse if taken with alcohol)
Miconazole 2% cream	Fungal foot/groin infections	Apply bd for 10 days	Local irritation, itching
Morphine (IM inj)	Severe pain	5–10mg IM every 2–4 h	Avoid with respiratory depression, head injury
Naloxone (IV inj)	Reversal of opiates in overdose	100–400mcg IV; repeat 200mcg inj every 2 minutes, as needed	May cause low or high blood pressure, heart arrhythmias, collapse. Use only under medical direction

Drug	Indication	Adult Dose	Common Side Effects
Ondansetron (tab under tongue)	Seasickness	4–8mg tds	Occasionally causes constipation
Oxycodone (SC inj or tab)	Severe pain	5–20mg SC every 4–6 h	Avoid with respiratory depression, head injury
Oxytocin + ergometrine	Antihaemorrhage from uterus (miscarriage)		Use only under the medical direction of a doctor
Paracetamol	Mild pain	1g qds	Not with other drugs containing paracetamol. Avoid with liver disease
Permethrin 1% cream rinse or 5% cream	Lice, scabies, and crab infestations	Apply to whole body, let dry; wash off after 12 h	Avoid contact with eyes, broken, infected skin
Phytomenadione (vit K1) pediatric IM injection	Routine injection for newborn	1 0.2ml amp IM once	Given after birth, IM or IV
Pilocarpine 2%	Treatment of glaucoma	Apply qds	Headache, blurred vision
Prednisolone	Anti-allergy	10–60mg od	May cause indigestion, abdominal discomfort
Prochlorperazine (IM inj)	Seasickness, other causes of sickness	12.5mg IM, then oral therapy 6 h later	May cause drowsiness, dry mouth, rarely tremor
Prochlorperazine (tab under tongue)	Seasickness	3mg tds	May cause drowsiness, dry mouth, rarely tremor
Prochlorperazine (tab)	Seasickness	10mg tds	May cause drowsiness, dry mouth, rarely tremor
Promethazine	Seasickness (antihistamine)	25mg every 6–8 h	Drowsiness (common); also urinary retention, dry mouth
Pseudoephedrine (tab)	Nasal decongestant	60mg qds	Anxiety, fast heart rate, difficulty sleeping
Ranitidine	Severe indigestion	150mg bd	May occasionally cause diarrhoea, stomach upset
Salbutamol (inhaler)	Asthma/wheeze	2 puffs qds or as needed	May cause tremor, fast heart rate, headache with frequent use
Silver sulfadiazine 1% cream	Prophylaxis; treatment of infection in burn wounds	Apply to wound od, more frequently if discharge	Allergic reactions—itch, rash, burning sensation; apply in sterile manner. Sun skin sensitivity
Tetracaine 1% eye drops	Anaesthesia for the eye	3–4 drops and wait several minutes	Stings the eye for a short time
Tramadol (IV or IM inj, or oral)	Moderate to severe pain	100mg every 4–6 h	Avoid with respiratory depression, head injury, epilepsy
Tranexamic acid (tab or IV inj)	Blood loss due to major trauma. Heavy periods (menorrhagia)	0.5–1g (more in trauma)	Use only under direction of a doctor
Trimethoprim	Urinary infections	200mg bd	May cause nausea, vomiting, itching
Tropicamide 1% eye drops	Dilation of the pupil for examination of the retina	3–4 drops	Stinging, irritation, blurred vision

PAIN RELIEF LADDER

Analgesics (painkillers) come in a variety of forms, work in different, often complementary, ways, and have different strengths. There are contraindications for using certain analgesics in certain people.

Combinations of differing types of analgesics are often effective in combatting pain. Therefore, one could take paracetamol and ibuprofen or diclofenac together, but not ibuprofen and diclofenac.

There is a "ladder" of pain relief, which is shown in the table below. Note that the same types of analgesics should not be taken together.

Name	Type	Severity of pain	Dose	Contra-indications
Paracetamol	Paracetamol	Mild to moderate pain	1g every 6 h	Previous allergy; not with other drugs containing paracetamol
Codydramol	Contains paracetamol	Mild to moderate pain	2 tablets every 6 h	Previous allergy; not with paracetamol
Aspirin	NSAID (Nonsteroidal anti-inflammatory)	Mild to moderate pain	Up to 900mg every 6 h	Previous allergy; stomach ulcers; asthma
Ibuprofen	NSAID	Mild to moderate pain	400mg every 4-6 h	Previous allergy; stomach ulcers, asthma
Diclofenac	NSAID	Moderate pain	75mg every 12 h 50mg every 8 h	Previous allergy; stomach ulcers; asthma
Dihydrocodeine	Opioid	Moderate to severe pain	40mg every 6 h	Previous allergy; respiratory depression; head injury
Methoxyflurane (Penthrox®)	Halogenated ether	Moderate to severe pain	Self-administered inhaler; 3–6ml per day. Avoid using on consecutive days	Renal or liver disease; diabetes; other nephrotoxic drugs
Tramadol	Opioid-like	Moderate to severe pain	100mg every 6 h	Previous allergy; respiratory depression; head injury; epilepsy
Morphine	Opioid	Severe pain	10mg IM inj every 2-4 h. If still in pain, seek medical advice	Previous allergy; respiratory depression; head injury

ANTIBIOTICS GUIDE

- ☐ If allergic to one antibiotic type, give another type and monitor closely.
- ☐ Many antibiotics may cause abdominal upset, and all antibiotics can cause allergic reactions (rash, swelling, collapse – see p.50).
- ☐ Antibiotics in tablet form are listed here, unless stated otherwise; check the medical kit for other preparations such as suppositories, injections etc.
- ☐ Check the information leaflet with the antibiotic for dosage and side effects.

Antibiotic	Type	Adult Dose	Notes (see medicine information leaflet)
Ear infections			
External ear infection			
Chloramphenicol drops		2–3 drops 2–3x/day	
Flucloxacillin	Penicillin	250–500mg 4x/day	Oral and IV preparations
Eye and ear drops	Mixed	2–3 drops 3x/day	Antibiotic/fungal/inflammatory
Middle ear infection			
Amoxicillin	Penicillin	250–500mg 3x/day	
Erythromycin	Macrolide	250–500mg 3x/day	May cause diarrhoea and vomiting
Doxycycline	Tetracycline	100mg 1x/day	Sun skin reaction, not for children
Eye infections			
Chloramphenicol drops		2–3 drops 2–3x/day	
Dental infections			
Amoxicillin + clavulanic acid	Penicillin	375–625mg 3x/day	Oral and IV preparations
Metronidazole	Nitroimidazole	400mg 3x/day	Sick if taken with alcohol
Chest infections			
Azithromycin	Macrolide	500mg 1x/day	
Amoxicillin + clavulanic acid	Penicillin	375–625mg 3x/day	Oral and IV preparations
Ceftriaxone	Cephalosporin	1–2g 1x/day injection	IV or IM
Doxycycline	Tetracycline	100mg 1x/day	Sun skin reaction, not for children
Abdominal infections			
Ciprofloxacin	Quinolone	250–500mg 2x/day	May cause tendonitis
Metronidazole	Nitroimidazole	400mg 3x/day	Sick if taken with alcohol
Ceftriaxone	Cephalosporin	1g 1x/day injection	IV or IM
Mebendazole	Benzimidazole	100mg 2x/day	For worm infections
Diarrhoea/Vomiting			
Ciprofloxacin	Quinolone	250–500mg 2x/day	May cause tendonitis
Metronidazole	Nitroimidazole	400mg 3x/day	Sick if taken with alcohol
Erythromycin	Macrolide	250–500mg 3x/day	May cause diarrhoea and vomiting
Genito-Urinary infections			
Ciprofloxacin	Quinolone	250–500mg 2x/day	May cause tendonitis
Amoxicillin + clavulanic acid	Penicillin	375–625mg 3x/day	Oral and IV preparations
Clotrimazole pessary	Imidazole	500mg pessary once	Vaginal irritation (fungal infection)
Trimethoprim	-	200mg 2x/day	May cause itching
Skin infections			
Fusidic acid	-	3–4x/day topical	
Flucloxacillin	Penicillin	250–500mg 4x/day	
Erythromycin	Macrolide	250–500mg 3x/day	May cause diarrhoea and vomiting
Miconazole	Imidazole	2x/day topical	Fungal groin/foot infections

HELICOPTER EVACUATION

- Evacuation by helicopter is a very costly resource and should be used wisely.
- Not without risk to boat and helicopter crew.
- Training exercises are invaluable; take advantage of any opportunity.
- The normal range for helicopter rescue is within 320 km (200 miles), occasionally using a fixed-wing plane to initially locate the boat.

Communicate
- Good communication with shore and helicopter crew is essential to ensure coordination and convey medical information regarding the victim.
- Brief your crew beforehand – it will be too noisy later.
- Communicate with the helicopter on VHF Ch 16.

Prepare
- Use gloves to avoid electrical shocks and rope burns.
- Clear the deck of loose objects. Clear the port stern quarter of obstructions.
- The victim should be dressed and ready (with medical record attached).
- All crew should wear lifejackets and be clipped to the boat.
- Use a bucket into which the initial weighted line (hi-line) will be coiled.

Position
- The boat should steer a straight course, close-hauled on port, with the helicopter hovering off to port (avoids downdraft hitting yacht).
- Motor or sail – with reduced sail –with enough speed to maintain steerage way.
- Rescue will usually take place from the starboard door of the helicopter and the port side of the boat.

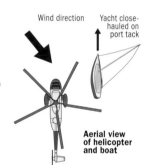

Wind direction   Yacht close-hauled on port tack

Aerial view of helicopter and boat

Method
- Do as the helicopter crew tell you – they are the experts.
- A hi-line is dropped from the helicopter. Do not touch it until it has earthed in the water or on the boat. Coil it into the bucket.
- DO NOT ATTACH THE LINE TO THE BOAT AND DO NOT LET IT GET SNAGGED.
- A winchman descends on the main lifting wire – pull the diver into the boat.
- Follow the winchman's directions.
- In rough weather, the casualty may be recovered from a life raft trailed astern or directly from the water. A single or double strop or a stretcher may be used.
- If necessary for indicating location, use a handheld red flare or orange smoke as a signal. Do not fire parachute or mini-flares when the helicopter is close by.

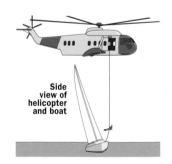

Side view of helicopter and boat

LIFE RAFT EVACUATION PROCEDURE

- ☐ Taking to the life raft must be the last resort; everything possible must be done to keep the boat afloat. It is said that crew should "step up" into a life raft.
- ☐ All crew should take an offshore survival course to both learn and experience the correct way to launch, inflate, right (if capsized), enter, and stabilize a life raft.
- ☐ Life rafts are heavy, particularly when packed in a canister, and must be readily accessible in the event of a sudden sinking. Life rafts stored on deck, in cradle-mounted canisters with hydrostatic release units, enable fast or automatic launching.

Communicate

- ☐ Brief the crew regularly on the procedure for abandoning ship and the storage location of the emergency equipment, the grab bag, and the life raft.
- ☐ When disaster strikes, stay calm, prioritize, communicate clearly with the crew, and allocate defined, achievable tasks.
- ☐ Institute a MAYDAY on the radio, and monitor Channel 16 or SSB 2182kHz.
- ☐ Activate an EPIRB and designate a crew member to take it onto the life raft.
- ☐ Launch a parachute flare if there is any chance of ships within range.

Prepare

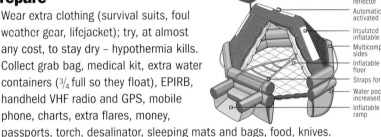

Features of a life raft
- Inflatable radar reflector
- Automatically activated light
- Insulated reflective inflatable canopy
- Multicompartment sides
- Inflatable insulated floor
- Straps for boarding
- Water pockets for increased stability
- Inflatable boarding ramp

- ☐ Wear extra clothing (survival suits, foul weather gear, lifejacket); try, at almost any cost, to stay dry – hypothermia kills.
- ☐ Collect grab bag, medical kit, extra water containers ($^3/_4$ full so they float), EPIRB, handheld VHF radio and GPS, mobile phone, charts, extra flares, money, passports, torch, desalinator, sleeping mats and bags, food, knives.
- ☐ Have a large drink of water, and take seasickness pills, even if you don't feel sick.

Method

- ☐ Attach the life raft painter to the boat SECURELY before moving the life raft around on a heaving deck – it may go over the side prematurely.
- ☐ Launch from the lee side into water clear of debris and give the painter a sharp tug.
- ☐ If the raft inflates upside down, try to right it from the boat – get into the water only as a last resort.
- ☐ Keep the raft close to the boat, especially in windy weather.
- ☐ Try to get in directly from the boat, but do not jump in – this may damage the floor
- ☐ Heaviest and strongest crew should get in first, to stabilize raft and help the injured
- ☐ Stay attached to the boat until it sinks. The larger vessel will be easier to see
- ☐ Once on board the raft, deploy the sea anchor, check the raft for damage, secure loose gear, check crew for injuries, issue seasickness tablets, and ration water.
- ☐ Insulate the raft floor by inflating it if possible, or using mats, sleeping bags etc.
- ☐ Close the door, but keep watch.
- ☐ Keep spirits up and be determined to survive and be rescued.

MAN OVERBOARD

Losing crew over the side is an ever-present risk that requires a calm, skilled response to effect a rapid recovery. This must be followed by a thorough, structured assessment of the casualty, particularly as sudden illness or injury may have caused the fall initially, or the casualty may have been injured while going over the side. Assessment should start with ABCDE (see p.32), followed by evaluation for prolonged immersion and drowning, trauma, and medical problems. Subsequently, especially in cases of near-drowning, the casualty may start to deteriorate, requiring medical support and urgent vacuation.

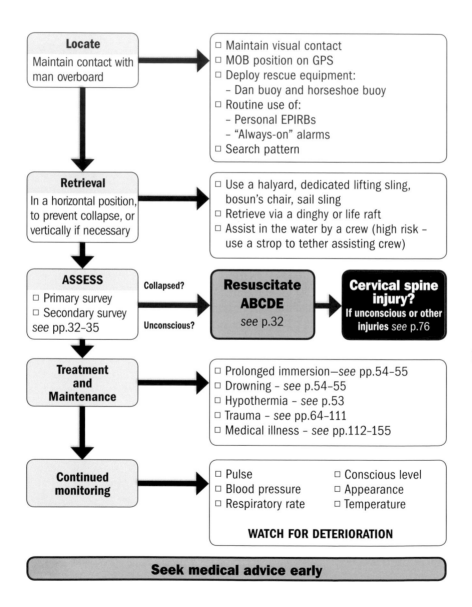

Locate
Maintain contact with man overboard

- Maintain visual contact
- MOB position on GPS
- Deploy rescue equipment:
  - Dan buoy and horseshoe buoy
- Routine use of:
  - Personal EPIRBs
  - "Always-on" alarms
- Search pattern

Retrieval
In a horizontal position, to prevent collapse, or vertically if necessary

- Use a halyard, dedicated lifting sling, bosun's chair, sail sling
- Retrieve via a dinghy or life raft
- Assist in the water by a crew (high risk – use a strop to tether assisting crew)

ASSESS
- Primary survey
- Secondary survey
see pp.32–35

Collapsed?

Unconscious?

Resuscitate ABCDE
see p.32

Cervical spine injury?
If unconscious or other injuries see p.76

Treatment and Maintenance

- Prolonged immersion—see pp.54–55
- Drowning – see p.54–55
- Hypothermia – see p.53
- Trauma – see pp.64–111
- Medical illness – see pp.112–155

Continued monitoring

- Pulse
- Blood pressure
- Respiratory rate
- Conscious level
- Appearance
- Temperature

WATCH FOR DETERIORATION

Seek medical advice early

DEALING WITH A DEATH ON-BOARD

Let me not pray to be sheltered from dangers but to be fearless in facing them.

Rabindranath Tagore, 1861-1941

Looking after the dying

Despite all efforts, sometimes you may be unable to prevent a casualty from dying. This is traumatic for all concerned, especially if you know or are related to the person or have been responsible for their treatment. But remember: even in an intensive care unit, patients sometimes die despite all possible treatments. Aboard a boat in the middle of the ocean, you have limited treatment options and can only do your best. Once you have accepted that the casualty will die, there is much you can do to ease the last few hours. It is a good idea to get medical advice if you are faced with someone who may be dying, and the next-of-kin should be informed.

Dignity Keep the casualty covered, replacing damaged or missing clothing. Obey any requests, if possible, and keep the casualty clean, as discreetly as possible.

Comfort The casualty's comfort, both physical and psychological, is imperative. Stay with the casualty continuously; make sure they know they are being cared for. Try to answer difficult questions, such as "Am I dying?", truthfully and with compassion. Make sure the casualty is comfortably positioned, warm, clean and dry. You may need comfort as well, from your crew mates.

Complete relief Aim for elimination of pain and suffering—if this cannot be achieved, seek medical advice. If simple painkillers are not enough, morphine will help to reduce pain and relieve mental anguish. It can be given as an intramuscular injection or intravenously if the casualty has vascular access. Give an antinausea drug (cyclizine) at the same time, because morphine may cause vomiting. Sedation, such as diazepam, can be given as well to reduce agitation—seek advice on dose and timing.

Communicate The casualty may not be able to talk properly, but they may wish to leave a message for loved ones. Make sure they know you understand and make a written record of their dying wishes. A second witness should sign and date it.

Signs of death

Take your time when trying to establish if the casualty is dead, and preferably do it with someone else. It can be very difficult in poorly lit conditions, in bad weather. Make a written record of time and place of death, and both sign the declaration. There are several body functions to assess when determining death:

Breathing Check that breathing has stopped. Listen, and feel with your cheek, very carefully over the mouth and nose. There should be no sign of chest or abdominal movement. Watch for a few minutes.

Heart Feel for the pulse over the carotid (*see* p.166). Listen with your ear to the chest over the heart or use a stethoscope. There should be no noise of the heart beating. Do these assessments for several minutes, longer if you are not sure.

Pupils The pupils will be very large and will not react to a bright light being shone into them.

Painful stimulus Pain provokes no reaction. Watch the face carefully when firmly squeezing the nail bed of both hands and rubbing firmly on the centre of the chest.

Mistakes when diagnosing death

Hypothermia Hypothermia may mimic death, especially if body temperature is less than 31°C. Take a rectal or oral temperature. If in any doubt, try to warm the casualty to above 31°C and reassess. The pulse may be very slow and weak and the breathing irregular and shallow (*see* p.53).

Drugs Certain drugs, particularly sedative drugs such as benzodiazepines and opiates, may cause the casualty to have a very weak and slow pulse, with shallow breathing. Seek medical advice if there is any suspicion of drugs being involved.

What to do after the death

Take some time after the death to look after yourself and your crewmates. The body should be cleaned and dried. Make sure the eyes are shut (tape might be needed), the hair neat and tidy, and the bladder empty (push on the lower abdomen). Bind the legs together at the ankles and interlock the fingers across the thighs. Maintain dignity by replacing clothes.

Record all details of:
□ The dead person, date of birth, address, next-of-kin
□ Circumstances leading up to the death (accident, illness, suspicious circumstances)
□ The body, including photographs of face, distinguishing marks, and injuries
□ All details of the clothing worn at the time of death—bag and keep them
□ All personal effects, which should be bagged, to be handed over to the authorities
□ All medical record charts
□ Time, place, and position of death
□ Statements from each of the crew regarding the circumstances of the death
□ Who assessed whether the person was dead
□ Any last wishes or messages from the dead person
□ Who provided medical advice.

What to do with the body

Ideally, the body should be kept and transported to shore as quickly as possible, to be handed over to the authorities. This may not be possible if the boat is weeks from port, in tropical climes. In colder oceans, the body should be placed in a body bag, if it is available, or wrapped tightly in sailcloth and sewn in securely. The body should be stored in as cold a place as possible, such as next to the hull in the bottom of the boat.

Burial at sea

If the body starts to decompose and becomes absolutely unbearable, burial at sea may be the only option. Make sure and document that the shore authorities know of your actions. The body should be placed in a shroud made from sailcloth and sewn in securely. A large weight should be placed in the shroud and a hole made to ensure the escape of gases of decomposition. An appropriate service should be performed, followed by a dignified committal of the body to the sea.

Record the time and position of the committal in the ship's log.

FURTHER RESOURCES

MAJOR AUTHORITIES

International Maritime Organization
www.imo.org
Maritime safety and environment protection.

World Sailing
www.sailing.org
Controlling authority of sailing throughout the world.

United Kingdom
Maritime and Coastguard Agency
www.mcga.gov.uk
Maritime safety and environment protection.

Australia/New Zealand
Australian Maritime Safety Authority
www.amsa.gov.au
Maritime qualifications and Search and Rescue.

Australian Volunteer Coast Guard Association
www.coastguard.com.au
Runs seamanship, marine radio, and navigation courses and co-ordinates Search and Rescue.

Maritime New Zealand
www.msa.govt.nz
Maritime safety and environment protection.

Yachting Australia
www.yachting.org.au
Governs the sport of yachting in Australia.

Yachting New Zealand
www.yachtingnz.org.nz
New Zealand's national body for competitive and recreational sailing.

MEDICAL SUPPORT AT SEA

United Kingdom
Medical Support Offshore
www.msos.org.uk
Medical kits, training, and support.

Yacht Lifeline
www.yachtlifeline.com
Medical services for the yachting industry.

TRAVEL ADVICE

World Health Organisation International Travel and Health
www.who.int/ith
News on the main health risks for travellers.

United Kingdom
MASTA Travel Clinics
www.masta-travel-health.com
Online health briefs and a network of travel clinics.

UK Department of Health Travel Health Advice
www.dh.gov.uk/en/Healthcare/Healthadvicefortravellers
Medical treatment abroad, health updates, information and advice on major diseases.

UK Foreign and Commonwealth Office Travel Advice
www.fco.gov.uk/en/travelling-and-living-overseas
Advice on staying safe and healthy abroad.

Australia/New Zealand
Australian Department of Foreign Affairs and Trade
www.smartraveller.gov.au
Advice, bulletins, and traveller registration.

NZ Ministry of Foreign Affairs and Trade
www.safetravel.govt.nz
Travel news and advice, including information on reciprocal healthcare agreements.

The Travel Doctor
www.traveldoctor.com.au
Travel medicine services, including dedicated clinics.

MEDICAL KIT SUPPLIERS

United Kingdom/Europe
Medical Support Offshore
www.msos.org.uk
Customised medical kits by expert physicians.

Australia/New Zealand
LFA First Response
www.lfafirstresponse.com.au
First aid products and basic marine kits.

First Aid Kits Australia
www.firstaidkitsaustralia.com.au
Medical supplies and equipment.

Safety at Sea
www.safetyatsea.co.nz
Advice on staying safe while at sea.

Pharmacy Direct
www.pharmacydirect.co.nz
Online pharmacy with first aid supplies.

BOOKS

Her Majesty's Department of Transport (HMDT). *Ship Captain's Medical Guide*, 22nd edn. Lanham, MD: Bernan Press, 2018.

World Health Organisation. *International Medical Guide for Ships*, 3rd edn. Switzerland: World Health Organisation Press, 2007.

INDEX

ACKNOWLEDGEMENTS

Front cover and chapter opener illustration: Cecilia Bandiera
All illustrations inside this book by Mark Franklin except for the following:
Page 67 top by Robert Brandt

This book is dedicated to our long-suffering wives, Miranda and Liz, with gratitude for their continued encouragement, support, and tolerance. Our thanks go to the many yachtsmen with whom we have sailed over the years, who have suffered our medical attentions uncomplainingly. We would like to pay tribute to Chay Blyth and Andrew Roberts, who knew the value of good, comprehensive medical support for yachtsmen. Finally, we would like to thank all of the staff at Marshall Editions. Their help and advice have been absolutely invaluable and their patience, legendary.

Spike Briggs
Campbell Mackenzie